SpringerBriefs in Applied Sciences and Technology

SpringerBriefs present concise summaries of cutting-edge research and practical applications across a wide spectrum of fields. Featuring compact volumes of 50–125 pages, the series covers a range of content from professional to academic.

Typical publications can be:

- A timely report of state-of-the art methods
- An introduction to or a manual for the application of mathematical or computer techniques
- A bridge between new research results, as published in journal articles
- A snapshot of a hot or emerging topic
- An in-depth case study
- A presentation of core concepts that students must understand in order to make independent contributions

SpringerBriefs are characterized by fast, global electronic dissemination, standard publishing contracts, standardized manuscript preparation and formatting guidelines, and expedited production schedules.

On the one hand, **SpringerBriefs in Applied Sciences and Technology** are devoted to the publication of fundamentals and applications within the different classical engineering disciplines as well as in interdisciplinary fields that recently emerged between these areas. On the other hand, as the boundary separating fundamental research and applied technology is more and more dissolving, this series is particularly open to trans-disciplinary topics between fundamental science and engineering.

Indexed by EI-Compendex, SCOPUS and Springerlink.

More information about this series at http://www.springer.com/series/8884

Fábio A. O. Fernandes · Ricardo J. Alves de Sousa
Mariusz Ptak

Head Injury Simulation
in Road Traffic Accidents

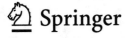 Springer

Fábio A. O. Fernandes
Center for Mechanical Technology and
 Automation (TEMA)
University of Aveiro
Aveiro
Portugal

Mariusz Ptak
Wrocław University of Science and
 Technology
Wrocław
Poland

Ricardo J. Alves de Sousa
Center for Mechanical Technology and
 Automation (TEMA)
University of Aveiro
Aveiro
Portugal

ISSN 2191-530X   ISSN 2191-5318 (electronic)
SpringerBriefs in Applied Sciences and Technology
ISBN 978-3-319-89925-1   ISBN 978-3-319-89926-8 (eBook)
https://doi.org/10.1007/978-3-319-89926-8

Library of Congress Control Number: 2018938647

Printed on acid-free paper

This Springer imprint is published by the registered company Springer International Publishing AG part of Springer Nature
The registered company address is: Gewerbestrasse 11, 6330 Cham, Switzerland

As humans, we can identify galaxies light years away; we can study particles smaller than an atom. But we still haven't unlocked the mystery of the three pounds of matter that sits between our ears.
—Barack Obama, *BRAIN Initiative inauguration, 2013.*

Acknowledgements

The authors gratefully acknowledge the Portuguese Foundation for Science and Technology (FCT) who financially supported this work through the scholarship SFRH/BD/91292/2012.

This publication was also developed as part of project LIDER/8/0051/L-8/ 16/NCBR/2017 funded by the National Centre for Research and Development, Poland.

Contents

1   **Finite Element Head Modelling and Head Injury Predictors**   1
    1.1   Head Injury Criteria and Thresholds   1
        1.1.1   Injury Criteria Based on Stresses and Strains
               in the Brain Tissue   4
    1.2   Finite Element Head Models 10
    References 16

2   **Development of a New Finite Element Human Head Model** 25
    2.1   Introduction 25
    2.2   Methods and Materials 27
        2.2.1   Geometric Modelling 27
        2.2.2   Description of the YEAHM 29
        2.2.3   Material Modelling 31
        2.2.4   Contact and Boundary Conditions 36
    References 36

3   **Validation of YEAHM** 41
    3.1   Simulation of Impacts on Cadavers 41
        3.1.1   Intracranial Pressure Response Validation 41
        3.1.2   Influence of Mesh Quality on the Results 46
        3.1.3   Brain Motion Validation 52
    References 57

4   **Application of Numerical Methods for Accident Reconstruction
    and Forensic Analysis** 59
    4.1   Introduction 59
    4.2   Vulnerable Road User Impact—Pedestrian Kinematics 60
    4.3   Case Study—Pedestrian Accident Analysis 64
        4.3.1   Audi TT Vehicle Measurement 69
        4.3.2   Material Testing and Verification 71

4.4   Finite Element Vehicle Model   75
4.5   MultiBody Dummy Model   77
4.6   Vehicle-to-Pedestrian Impact Configuration   78
4.7   Analysis of the Results   81
4.8   Head to Windshield Impact   84
      4.8.1   Geometry Acquisition   85
      4.8.2   Boundary Conditions   87
      4.8.3   Windshield Modeling   89
      4.8.4   Analysis of the Results for Head-to-Windshield
              Impact—Biomechanical Perspective   94
4.9   Conclusions   95
References   96

Acronyms

ASDH	Acute subdural haematoma
AIS	Abbreviated injury scale
CAD	Computer-aided design
CAE	Computer-aided engineering
CNS	Central nervous system
COG	Centre of gravity
CPU	Central processing unit
CSDM	Cumulative strain damage measure
CSF	Cerebrospinal fluid
CT	Computer tomography
DAI	Diffuse axonal injury
DDM	Dilatation damage measure
EPP	Expanded polypropylene
EU	European Union
Euro NCAP	European New Car Assessment Programme
FE	Finite element
FEA	Finite element analysis
FEHM	Finite element head model
FEM	Finite element method
GHBMC	Global human body models consortium
HIC	Head injury criterion
HIP	Head impact power
KTH	Kungliga Tekniska Högskolan
MADYMO	MAthematical DYnamic MOdeling
MRI	Magnetic resonance imaging
MTBI	Mild traumatic brain injury
NURBS	Non-uniform rational basis spline
PMHS	Post-Mortem Human Subjects
PVB	Polyvinyl butyral
RMDM	Relative motion damage measure

ROI	Region of interest
SDH	Subdural haematoma
SIMon	SImulated injury Monitor
STL	STereoLithography
SUFEHM	Strasbourg University FEHM
SUV	Sports utility vehicle
TBI	Traumatic brain injury
THUMS	Total human model for safety
TTC	Time to collision
TTD	Time to decision
UCDBTM	University College Dublin Brain Trauma Model
VRU	Vulnerable road users
WAD	Wrap around distance
WFD	Waveform digitizing technology
WSUHIM	Wayne State University Head Injury Model
YEAHM	YEt another head model

Chapter 1
Finite Element Head Modelling and Head Injury Predictors

1.1 Head Injury Criteria and Thresholds

First, it is important to highlight the terminology used in this book related to head/brain injuries. General public more readily associate the negative symptoms to "brain injury" (judged as more serious) rather than to "head injury" (less serious, in their view), despite the fact the description may be related to the same injury event (McKinlay 2011). The authors of this book will use the terms head/brain injury interchangeably regarding brain injury. Head injury refers to any damage caused to its contents, for instance a skull fracture or a skin laceration.

The cerebral cortex is the largest and most complex part of the brain. It consists of left and right hemispheres, which are interconnected by means of the corpus callosum. These hemispheres are divided into four lobes—frontal, parietal, temporal and occipital (Fig. 1.1).

Under the cerebral cortex is the white matter. The diencephalon connects the brain with brainstem, which includes the midbrain, the core and the pons (Andaluz 2016). In the brainstem there are centres that are responsible for the coordination of functions such as blood circulation, breathing and consciousness (Aare 2003). The cerebellum is in the back of the head and consist of two hemispheres (Andaluz 2016).

A common result from traffic accidents are injuries to the middle meningeal artery. The patient within 30 minutes of injury may not feel any discomfort, yet arterial bleeding leads to detachment of the dura from the cranial vault, resulting in an epidural hematoma (Aare 2003). These and other effects of brain injuries are presented in Table 1.1.

Head injury typically results from either a direct impact to the head or from an indirect force applied to the head-neck system, when the torso is rapidly accelerated or decelerated. For both cases, the head sustains a combination of linear and rotational acceleration (Aare 2003). Generally, translational acceleration creates intracranial pressure gradients, while rotational acceleration rotates the skull relatively to the brain (Bandak 1997a).

For over half a century, research has been undertaken to assess plausible injury mechanisms causing inertial head injury during impact and to establish associated human head tolerance levels. The development of injury criteria has been a major goal

© The Author(s) 2018
F. A. O. Fernandes et al., *Head Injury Simulation in Road Traffic Accidents*, SpringerBriefs in Applied Sciences and Technology, https://doi.org/10.1007/978-3-319-89926-8_1

Fig. 1.1 The brain regions
and their vital functions
(Adapted from Andaluz
2016 and Aare 2003)

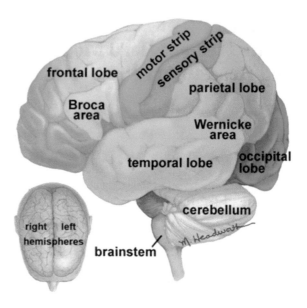

Table 1.1 Relation between symptoms and injured brain regions (Thamburaj 2012)

Brain region	Function	Symptom
Frontal lobe	Personality; Intelligence; Attention; Judgment; Body movement; Problem solving; Speech	Loss of movement (paralysis); Repetition of a single thought; Unable to focus on a task; Mood swings,irritability,impulsiveness Changes in social behaviour and personality; Difficulty with problem solving; Aphasia
Temporal lobe	Speech; Memory; Hearing; Sequencing; Organisation	Aphasia; Difficulty recognising faces; Difficulty identifying objects; Problems with memory; Changes in sexual behaviour; Increased aggressive behaviour
Occipital lobe	Vision	Defects in vision or blind spots; Blurred vision; Hallucinations; Difficulty reading and writing
Parietal lobe	Sense of touch, pain and temperature; Distinguishing size, shape and colour; Spatial and visual perception	Difficulty distinguishing left from right; Lack of awareness; Difficulties with eye-hand coordination; Problems reading and writing; Difficulty with mathematics
Cerebellum	Balance and coordination	Difficulty coordinating and walking; Tremors; Vertigo; Slurred speech
Brainstem	Breathing; Heart rate; Alertness/consciousness	Changes in breathing; Difficulty swallowing; Problems with balance and movement; Vertigo

among researchers in order to accurately evaluate the risk of sustaining a head injury and to assess the effectiveness of potential protective head gear such as helmets.

In fact, this is still an active area of research and scientists are trying to relate this type of damage with parameters such as forces or accelerations. This may provide a strong basis for improvements in restraint systems design. Head injury criteria can be roughly divided into three categories, as proposed by van den Bosch (2006):

- Injury criteria based on translational or rotational accelerations of the head's COG,
- Injury criteria based on translational and rotational accelerations of the head's COG,
- Injury criteria based on stresses and strains in the brain tissue.

Currently, many studies have presented thresholds to assess injury occurrence. A thorough review on head injury predictors and their respective thresholds was performed in Fernandes and Alves de Sousa (2015). In this chapter, only injury criteria based on parameters such as stresses and strains in the brain are addressed since these are typically used with finite element head models (FEHMs).

The referred types of injury criteria were mainly proposed considering closed head injury. Localised loads, which could be considered suitable criteria for skull fracture, depend on the impactor shape and skull thickness at the impact site. Table 1.2 presents a summary of fracture peak forces at different regions of the skull.

Hume et al. (1995) stated that a depressed skull fracture is likely to appear at the temporal area if the impacted area is less than 5 cm^2 and the pressure exceeds 4 MPa. McElhaney et al. (1970), Melvin et al. (1970) and Robbins and Wood (1969)

Table 1.2 Peak force for fracture at different regions of the skull

Impact area	Force [kN]	Reference
Frontal	4.0	Schneider and Nahum (1972)
	4.2	Nahum et al. (1968)
	4.3–4.5	Yoganandan et al. (1994)
	4.7	Allsop et al. (1988)
	5.5	Hodgson and Thomas (1971)
	6.2	Advani et al. (1975)
	15.6	Voo et al. (1994)
Temporal	2.0	Schneider and Nahum (1972)
	3.4–4.4	Yoganandan et al. (1994)
	3.6	Nahum et al. (1968)
	5.2	Allsop et al. (1991)
	6.2	Voo et al. (1994)
Occipital	11.7–11.9	Yoganandan et al. (1994)
	12.5	Advani et al. (1982)
Parietal	3.5	Hume et al. (1995)
Vertex	3.5	Yoganandan et al. (1994)

have reported cranial bone stress thresholds. According to the mentioned references, a compact cranial bone breaks in tension at 48–128 MPa, while the cancellous bone breaks in compression at 32–74 MPa. Raul et al. (2006) proposed a global strain energy of 2.2 J as a 50% risk indicator for skull fracture. Recently, Monea et al. (2014) suggested an energy failure level of 22–24 J for the frontal site and 5–15 J for the temporal region.

1.1.1 Injury Criteria Based on Stresses and Strains in the Brain Tissue

There is a tendency among researchers to use head injury predictors that are based on the head tissue level response, rather than on its kinematics. Brain injury is reported to correlate well with stress, strain and strain rate (Lee and Haut 1989; Viano and Lövsund 1999). However, strains and strain rates inside the brain are difficult to measure (van den Bosch 2006). This can be achieved using anatomical detailed and accurate FEHMs, where stresses and strains are used to compute injury parameters in the skull and in the intracranial contents. Therefore, these models bring a detailed injury assessment closer to reality, since they enable stresses and strains to be examined.

DiMasi et al. (1995) and Bandak (1995, 1997b) developed three component-level injury predictors representing the general types of brain injuries: the cumulative strain damage measure (CSDM), the dilatation damage measure (DDM) and the relative motion damage measure (RMDM). Other predictors have been proposed, such as the brain pressure tolerance and the brain von Mises stress and also strain.

More recently, Takhounts et al. (2003, 2008) proposed the SIMon FE model criteria based on the above-mentioned injury metrics proposed by DiMasi et al. (1995) and Bandak (1995, 1997b). Similarly, other FEHMs have their own specific criteria and thresholds. This is the case of Strasbourg University FEHM (SUFEHM) criteria, which is also reviewed in the this chapter. The following subsections cover the mentioned head injury criteria and their specific thresholds.

1.1.1.1 Brain Pressure

This is a head injury predictor based on the intracranial pressure. Several studies were published with thresholds for this predictor. Some are presented in Table 1.3.

Liu and Fan (1998), by using a FEHM, concluded that brain pressure has a better sensitivity for very short time impacts than the head injury criterion (HIC). However, computed brain pressure does not correlate with some brain injuries. Kang et al. (1997) and Miller et al. (1998) criticised this criterion's capability to predict brain injuries, particularly diffuse axonal injury (DAI). In addition, Willinger and Baumgartner (2003b) established that computed brain pressure is not correlated with the occurrence of brain haemorrhages, whereas brain von Mises stress is.

Table 1.3 Brain pressure thresholds

Brain injury	Pressure [kPa]	Reference
Moderate	172.3	Nahum et al. (1977)
Severe or fatal	234.4	
Minor or absent	$\leq$173	Ward and Chan (1980)
Severe (coup)	235	(Ward et al. 1980 and Chafi et al. 2009)
Severe (contrecoup)	$-$186	Ward et al. (1980)
Contusions, oedema and haematoma	200	(Willinger et al. 1999b; Baumgartner 2001) and Raul et al. (2006)
Coup	180	Yao et al. (2006)
AIS3+ (coup)	256	Yao et al. (2008)
AIS3+ (contrecoup)	$-$152	
50% risk of MTBI (coup)	90	Zhang et al. (2004)
50% risk of MTBI (contrecoup)	$-$76	

1.1.1.2 Brain von Mises Stress

This criterion assumes that the von Mises stress is the cause of brain damage. Some of the proposed thresholds are given in Table 1.4.

1.1.1.3 Cumulative Strain Damage Measure

This method was presented by Bandak and Eppinger (1994) to evaluate the strain-related damage within the brain. The idea behind their hypothesis is the possibility to quantify the mechanical damage in the axonal components of the brain, once the responsible state of strain is characterised.

Therefore, a cumulative damage measure based on the brain's cumulative volume fraction calculation, which has experienced a specific level of stretch (maximum principal strain) is used as a possible predictor for deformation-related brain injury such as DAI (Marjoux et al. 2008; Takhounts et al. 2008; Zhang et al. 2007).

The cumulative strain damage measure (CSDM) is based on the hypothesis that DAI is associated with the cumulative volume fraction (%) of the brain matter experiencing tensile strains over a critical level. At each time increment, the volume of all elements that have experienced a principal strain above prescribed threshold values is calculated. The affected brain volume monotonically increases in time during conditions where the brain is undergoing tensile stretching deformations, and remains constant for all other conditions (compression, unloading, etc). Bandak et al. (2001) found that a CSDM level 5 corresponds to mild DAI and a CSDM level of 22 corresponds to moderate-to-severe DAI, which means that 5% and 22% represent

Table 1.4 Stress thresholds

Brain injury	Stress [kPa]	Reference
TBI	11	Zhou et al. (1996)
	12	Yao et al. (2006)
	8 (in the temporal lobes)	Willinger et al. (1999b)
MTBI	50% probability: 18	Willinger and Baumgartner (2003a, b)
Severe TBI	16	Kang et al. (1997)
	27	Anderson (2000)
	46	Baumgartner et al. (2001)
	50% probability: 38	Willinger and Baumgartner (2003a, b)
Concussion	22	Baumgartner et al. (2001)
	20	Willinger et al. (2000a)
	40	Deck et al. (2003)
	Long duration: 20	COST327 (2001)
	Short duration: 10	
	50% probability: 8.4 (in the corpus callosum)	Kleiven (2007)
	50% probability: 7.8 (in the brainstem)	Zhang et al. (2004)
	50% probability: 18	Willinger and Baumgartner (2003a)
Mild DAI	50% probability: 26	Deck and Willinger (2008)
Severe DAI	50% probability: 33	
DAI	50% probability: 61.6	Sahoo et al. (2016)
AIS3+	14.8	Yao et al. (2008)

respectively the brain volume experiencing strain in excess relative to the critical level of 15%, proposed by Thibault et al. (1990). Takhounts et al. (2003) predicted a 50% probability of concussion for 55% of brain volume experiencing a 15% strain level. Later, Takhounts et al. (2008) predicted a 50% probability of DAI for 54% of brain volume experiencing a maximum principal strain of 0.25. Recently, as a 50% risk threshold for DAI, Sahoo et al. (2016) reported CSDM values of 0.85, 0.59 and 0.27 for strains of 0.10, 0.15 and 0.25, respectively.

Other proposed values of brain strain critical levels are presented in Table 1.5. The CSDM is often considered the most promising stress and strain based injury criterion, since it is based on the brain's tissue strain. This is an important parameter, mainly when the brain is submitted to considerable rotations that cause large strains, causing brain injuries such as DAI (Aare et al. 2003).

Table 1.5 Strain thresholds

Injury type	Threshold	Reference
Contusion	50% risk: 0.19 (in the cortex)	Shreiber et al. (1997)
	0.15 (in the cortex)	Thibault et al. (1990)
DAI	0.1	Thibault (1993)
	0.21	Bain and Meaney (2000)
	0.18	Wright and Ramesh (2012)
	0.2	Morrison III et al. (2003) and Kleiven (2007a)
	moderate-to-severe: 0.05-0.10	Margulies and Thibault (1992)
	50% probability of mild: 0.31	Deck and Willinger (2008)
	50% probability of severe: 0.4	
	50% probability: 0.21 (in the corpus callosum) 0.26 (in the grey matter)	Kleiven (2007)
	0.16	Singh et al. (2006)
	0.22	Nakadate et al. (2014)
	50% probability: 0.22	Sahoo et al. (2016)
MTBI	0.35–0.45	Viano et al. (2005)
	25% probability: 0.26 (in the midbrain)	Zhang et al. (2003)
	50% probability: 0.37 (in the midbrain)	
	75% probability: 0.49 (in the midbrain)	
Concussion	AIS1: 0.3 and AIS2: 0.35	Zhang et al. (2008)
	50% probability: 0.19 (in the midbrain)	Zhang et al. (2004)
	0.1	Kleiven (2007a)
	50% probability: 0.13 (in the thalamus) 0.15 (in the corpus callosum) 0.26 (in the white matter)	Patton et al. (2013)

1.1.1.4 Dilatation Damage Measure

The dilatation damage measure (DDM) is a pressure-based injury criterion proposed by Bandak (1997b), which evaluates brain injury caused by large dilatational stresses. It is supposed to correlate with contusions (Marjoux et al. 2008; Takhounts et al. 2008; Zhang et al. 2007), by monitoring the cumulative volume fraction of the brain experiencing specified negative pressure levels.

The DDM is similar to the brain pressure criterion presented previously. Nevertheless, this one focuses on the amount of dilatational damage caused by negative pressures, usually associated with contrecoup contusions. The probability of contusion is correlated with the brain volume fraction where negative pressures can produce damage (Vezin and Verriest 2004).

Similarly to the CSDM calculation, at each time step, the volume of all elements experiencing a negative pressure level exceeding a prescribed threshold value is calculated. Bandak et al. (2001) suggested a DDM value of 5% at a threshold level of -101 kPa as an injury threshold. Takhounts et al. (2003) predicted a 50% probability of contusion for a DDM value of 7.2% for a pressure of -100 kPa.

Other researchers have been presenting tolerance values for negative pressures. Ward et al. (1980) proposed a value of -186 kPa in tension as a brain tolerance limit. Zhang et al. (2004) proposed a value of -76 kPa as a 50% risk of mild traumatic brain injury (MTBI). Yao et al. (2006) proposed a critical value for contrecoup pressure of -130 kPa. More recently, Yao et al. (2008) presented a critical value for contrecoup pressure of -152 kPa as a predictor for AIS3+ injuries.

1.1.1.5   Relative Motion Damage Measure

The relative motion damage measure (RMDM) was proposed by Bandak (1997b) to evaluate injuries related to brain movements located at the inner surface of the cranium. RMDM monitors the brain surface tangential motion resulting from combined rotational and translational head accelerations. Such motions are suspected to be the cause of subdural haematoma (SDH) associated with large-stretch ruptures of the bridging veins (Marjoux et al. 2008), due to the brain motion relative to the skull.

The bridging veins have been described by Lee and Haut (1989) as having an ultimate strain of about 0.5 in tension, while Löwenhielm (1974) observed failure at strain values ranging from 0.2 to about 1, depending on the strain rate. A smaller range of 0.3–0.6, but still within the range observed by Löwenhielm (1974), was proposed by Monson et al. (2003) and Morrison III et al. (2003). Takhounts et al. (2003) proposed rupture of the bridging veins for a tolerance limit of 1. More recently, Monea et al. (2014) presented a critical value of 5 mm elongation or 25% stretch limit for the occurrence of acute subdural haematoma (ASDH) due to bridging veins rupture.

The majority of FEHMs do not have bridging veins. Nevertheless, RMDM does not require the modelling of the bridging veins, but rather the monitoring of the relative displacement between node pairs. Each pair represents a bridging vein tethered between the skull and the brain. Thus, RMDM relies heavily on the correct modelling of the interface between brain and skull. If the interface is modelled correctly, the RMDM is potentially a suitable injury criterion to predict SDH (Marjoux et al. 2008; Takhounts et al. 2008).

1.1.1.6   FEHMs Specific Criteria

Numerical head models can be useful tools to reconstruct accidents and even to assess protective head gear. In accordance with this line of thought, some research groups developed injury specific criteria to their models. The simulated injury monitor (SIMon), proposed by Takhounts et al. (2003), is one of these models. It was originally developed by DiMasi et al. (1995) and later improved by Bandak et al. (2001). More recently, this model was updated by Takhounts et al. (2008), presenting a new FEHM that comprised several parts: rigid skull, cerebrum, cerebellum, falx, tentorium, combined pia-arachnoid complex with cerebrospinal fluid (CSF), ventricles, brainstem, and parasagittal blood vessels. The model's topology was derived from human computer tomography (CT). The skull was assumed to be rigid, whereas the rest of the structures were considered as deformable, linear viscoelastic, isotropic, and homogeneous.

The SIMon crteria correspond to a set of thresholds obtained through reconstruction of real head impacts. These reconstructions were performed by Takhounts et al. (2003, 2008) and the predicted thresholds were already presented in the previous subsections. For instance, a 50% probability of concussion was predicted for:

- a CSDM value of 55% of brain volume experiencing a 15% strain level;
- a DDM value of 7.2% for a pressure of -100 kPa;

In addition, Takhounts et al. (2003) proposed rupture of the bridging veins for a tolerance limit of 1. More recently, Takhounts et al. (2008) predicted a 50% probability of DAI for:

- a CSDM value of 54% of brain volume experiencing a maximum principal strain of 0.25;
- any brain volume experiencing a maximum principal strain value of 0.87;

Similarly to SIMon criteria, SUFEHM has specific thresholds predicted by reconstructing real head impacts with injurious outcomes. As described in Willinger and Baumgartner (2003b), three injury criteria are computed with this model:

- The maximum von Mises stress value reached by a significant volume of at least 10 contiguous elements (representing about 3 cm^3 of brain volume) is proposed as a correlation to neurological injury occurrences. Marjoux et al. (2008), for a moderate and severe neurological injury, obtained von Mises stress values of 27 kPa and 39 kPa, respectively. More recently, Deck and Willinger (2009) updated these tolerance limits to 28 kPa and 53 kPa, respectively;
- The maximum value reached by the global internal strain energy of the elements modelling the space between the brain and skull is proposed as a correlation to SDH. This value represents the integral of $\sigma \times \varepsilon$ product over the whole domain between the brain and skull. Marjoux et al. (2008) found a maximum value reached by the global strain energy of the subarachnoidal space and proposed it as a correlation to SDH with a value of about 4211 mJ. This is higher than the 4 J proposed by COST327 (2001) as strain energy in the CSF, for prediction of SDH. More recently, Deck and Willinger (2009) updated this tolerance limit to 4950 mJ and proposed a CSF pressure of 290 kPa as tolerance for SDH;
- The maximum value reached by the global internal strain energy of the deformable skull is proposed as a correlation to skull fracture occurrences. Marjoux et al.

(2008) found an internal energy of 833 mJ. A lower value for strain energy magnitude (544 mJ) was proposed by Sahoo et al. (2013) as threshold for 50% risk of human skull bone fracture. More recently, this value was updated to 448 mJ (Sahoo et al. 2014b).

In addition, Deck and Willinger (2008, 2009) proposed a rational approach in order to evaluate the ability of head models to predict brain pressures and strains by using a statistical approach, predicting the following thresholds for DAI:

- Brain von Mises stress of 28 kPa for mild DAI and 53 kPa for severe DAI;
- Brain first principal strain of 33% for mild DAI and 67% for severe DAI.

All of these predictors are associated with an injury risk of 50%. More recently, the von Mises stress was updated to 61.6 kPa and the first principal strain to 0.93 for a 50% risk of severe DAI (Sahoo et al. 2016). Marjoux et al. (2008) assessed and compared the injury prediction capability of the HIC, the Head Impact Power (HIP) and the criteria provided by the SIMon FEHM and SUFEHM. Marjoux et al. (2008) found better injury predictions with SUFEHM criteria than SIMon criteria, justifying it with the simplicity of SIMon model, whereas SUFEHM geometry seems closer to the real head anatomy. This was also suggested by Franklyn et al. (2003), by comparing the results obtained with other state-of-the-art FEHM, the Wayne State University head injury model (WSUHIM), with the SIMon model.

Throughout this section, it was evident that there is a wide range of tolerance levels for each injury criterion that can be justified by different models: physical head models, FE models, animal models, clinical and cadaver models (Hrapko et al. 2008; Wright and Ramesh 2012). Over the years, with the increasing CPU power, FEM appears to be one of the most useful tools for researchers in this field. Once a FEHM is validated and the proper criteria are settled, it may be used to predict accurately the injury outcome from head impacts. During the last decade, complex FEHMs have been developed. In the next section, these are reviewed.

1.2 Finite Element Head Models

Over the years, FEHMs have been used to understand and predict the head response under several impact conditions. These models allow an accurate computational-based prediction of brain injuries, by relating the results to medical investigations based on autopsies of corpses involved in real accidents (Kang et al. 1997). Nowadays, with the huge development of CPU power, head modelling has evolved tremendously.

Nowadays, only 3D models are relevant for most impact analysis. Nevertheless, 2D models are still used for parametric studies of controlled planar motions (Darvish and Crandall 2002; Wright and Ramesh 2012). Indeed, since a long time ago, there is a great interest in FE models for head injury research. One of the first 3D models was developed by Ward and Thompson (1975). This is a simple model, with simplified geometries and linear material properties. Later, Shugar (1977) developed a 3D model, by upgrading a previous 2D version (Shugar and Katona 1975). In the same year, other simplified models were developed (Khalil and Hubbard 1977; Nahum et al. 1977).

A few years later, a great step was made by Hosey and Liu (1982), presenting a geometric improved FEHM with brain and neck. Over the years, more FEHMs had been presented, always with complexer geometries (DiMasi et al. 1991; Mendis 1992; Ruan et al. 1991). In fact, Krabbel and Müller (1996) and Hartmann and Kruggel (1999) developed a FEHM using CT and magnetic resonance imaging (MRI) scans to model the skull and brain geometries.

At this point, some of the current state-of-the-art FEHMs were firstly presented. For instance, the first version of WSUHIM (Ruan et al. 1993; Zhou et al. 1995, 1996). This one was already capable of differentiating the material properties between grey and white matter. The second version of WSUHIM was developed and upgraded by Al-Bsharat et al. (1999), by introducing a sliding interface between skull and brain.

More recently, the final version of WSUHIM (Fig. 1.2), was presented by Zhang et al. (2001). This includes scalp, skull, dura, falx cerebri, tentorium, CSF and brain with distinct white and grey matter. Concerning the mechanical properties, the brain is characterised as viscoelastic and an elastic-plastic material model was used for bone.

This model was validated against cadaveric intracranial and ventricular pressure data (Nahum et al. 1977), relative brain/skull displacement data (Hardy et al. 2001), and facial impact data (Trosseille et al. 1992). It was also validated against pedestrian accidents data (Dokko et al. 2003). In addition, it was used to reconstruct 53 cases of sport accidents including 22 cases of concussion by King et al. (2003).

Another model was developed by Claessens et al. (1997), which includes skull, brain and dura mater. This model was validated for intracranial pressure, by simu-

Fig. 1.2 Wayne State University brain injury model (WSUHIM) (adapted from Zhang et al. 2001)

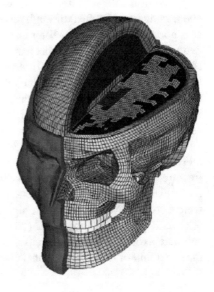

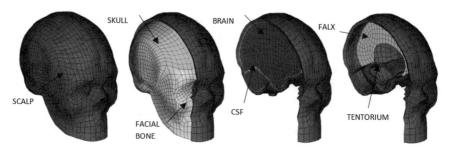

Fig. 1.3 SUFEHM (adapted from Fernandes et al. 2013)

lating the cadaver experiments of Nahum et al. (1977). Later, Brands et al. (2002) upgraded this model, by incorporating nonlinear material behaviour on the brain response. Nevertheless, all structures were assumed to be rigidly connected to each other.

Also in the 90s, Kang et al. (1997) presented a FEHM that is currently considered a state-of-the-art model, called SUFEHM. The external geometry of the skull was digitised from a human adult male and the interior geometry was obtained from an atlas. This model also includes other anatomical features such as the scalp, dura matter and brain, as shown in Fig. 1.3. Viscoelastic properties were assigned to the brain and the other features were modelled as isotropic and homogenous (Khalil and Viano 1982). This model was validated (Willinger et al. 1999a, b, 2000c), with regard to cadaveric experiments (Hardy et al. 2001; Nahum et al. 1977; Trosseille et al. 1992; Yoganandan et al. 1994, 1995). More details about the development and validation of this model are described in Willinger et al. (2000a, b), Willinger and Baumgartner (2003a) and Deck and Willinger (2009).

In addition, tolerance limits were identified by Marjoux et al. (2008) and Willinger and Baumgartner (2003a) through reconstruction of real accidents, being recognised as a good DAI predictor (Miller et al. 1998; Smith et al. 2003). However, a well-defined correlation between mechanical loading and DAI using FEHM has not been achieved yet (Cloots et al. 2010). A possible contribution to this is that the gyri and sulci in the brain, which are not included in the actual FEHM, can play an important role in the local tissue deformations (Cloots et al. 2008; Lauret et al. 2009). Ho and Kleiven (2009) suggested that the inclusion of sulci should be considered in FEHM as it alters the strain and strain distribution.

More recently, Sahoo et al. (2013, 2014b) upgraded SUFEHM, by developing a more realistic skull geometry with a variable thickness, which is able to simulate skull fracture. This one was used to reconstruct real-world trauma accidents, developing a new skull fracture criterion (Sahoo et al. 2016b). The brain mechanical properties were also improved, focusing on high strain rates and nonlinear behaviour (Nicolle et al. 2004). Later, Sahoo et al. (2014) upgraded the model in order to be able to simulate axonal elongation in cases of head trauma. This was validated, showing the feasibility of integrating axonal direction information into FEHMs. This recently

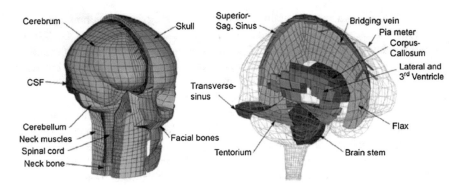

Fig. 1.4 KTH FEHM (adapted from Ho and Kleiven 2007)

upgraded model was used to develop new predictors for DAI, by reconstructing 109 head trauma cases (Sahoo et al. 2016).

Another state-of-the-art model is the Kungliga Tekniska Högskolan (KTH) human head model presented in Fig. 1.4. This model was developed by Kleiven (2002) and comprises nonlinear viscoelastic, incompressible material modelling. It includes scalp, skull, brain, meninges, CSF and 11 pairs of parasagittal bridging veins. A simplified neck was also modelled.

The KTH model has been validated (Kleiven and Hardy 2002; Kleiven and von Holst 2001, 2002) against experimental pressure data (Nahum et al. 1977; Trosseille et al. 1992) and relative motion data (Hardy et al. 2001). More recently, it was also validated against intracerebral acceleration experiments (Kleiven 2006b) and skull fracture experiments (Kleiven 2006a). Kleiven (2007) compared various predictors for MTBI, reconstructing real-world accidents.

Ho and Kleiven (2007) studied the influence of including vasculature in the KTH model by modelling a set of blood vessels and concluded that it could be useful for studying ASDH, since ruptures can be predicted by measuring the strain directly in the blood vessels. Later, Ho and Kleiven (2009) studied and suggested the inclusion of sulci in FEHMs, since it alters the strain and stresses distribution in an FE model. In other studies, it is also suggested that the folding structure of the brain surface and the non-uniform distribution of the CSF greatly influence both the distribution and the magnitude of the maximum stress and strains in the brain (Cloots et al. 2008; Gilchrist and O'Donoghue 2000; Lauret et al. 2009). The KTH model suffered some modifications to be used in some specific studies, such as the changes done by Li et al. (2011) in order to model the ventricular system. More recently, the influence of anisotropy was included in this model (Giordano et al. 2014), by modelling the neural fibres and thus including the axonal orientation as in SUFEHM (Sahoo et al. 2014, 2016).

Another model, the University College Dublin Brain Trauma Model (UCDBTM), based on CT and MRI data, was developed by Horgan and Gilchrist (2003), being improved later by Horgan and Gilchrist (2004). The model comprises a scalp, skull, dura, CSF, falx, tentorium and brain. This was validated against intracranial pressure data from Nahum et al. (1977) and brain motion data from Hardy et al. (2001). Further validations were accomplished, comparing real-world brain injury events to model reconstructions (Doorly and Gilchrist 2006). More recently, Yan and Pangestu (2011) improved UCDBTM by including viscoelasticity in the material definition of almost all tissues. In addition, CSF was modelled as a hydrostatic fluid.

In the last decade, several new models were presented. After state-of-the-art models, such as WSUHIM, KTH, SUFHEM and UCDBTM, being developed, the majority of these new models did not improve or bring something new. Most of them have oversimplified geometries and material properties, being modelled with linear elastic models, with rigid connected parts or were not properly validated (Belingardi et al. 2005; Cardamone 2005; Dirisala et al. 2011; Kim et al. 2005; Motherway et al. 2009; Suh et al. 2005; Ziejewski et al. 2009). From this point, only some models are worth mentioning. For instance, the SIMon model developed by Takhounts et al. (2008) and already presented in Sect. 1.1.1.6.

Canaple et al. (2003) developed a new model, focusing on the representation of the skull/brain interface and using a hyperelastic material to represent the CSF. Nevertheless, the material properties assigned to the other parts were isotropic and homogeneous. This model was validated for the cadaver impact tests of Nahum et al. (1977) and used in accidents reconstruction (Canaple et al. 2002).

A 3D model of the head-neck complex has been developed by Kimpara et al. (2006) including a detailed description of the brain and the spinal cord. According to the authors, the brain-spinal cord model was useful to investigate the central nervous system (CNS) injuries. This model was validated against three sets of brain test data (Hardy et al. 2001; Nahum et al. 1977; Trosseille et al. 1992). In the same year, Yao et al. (2006) presented a FEHM that includes the main anatomical head structures, such as CSF, meninges and brain. This model was validated for Nahum et al. (1977) tests, and then used to reconstruct real-world pedestrian accidents (Yao et al. 2008; Yang 2011).

Iwamoto et al. (2002) presented a FEHM that includes a skull, CSF, sagittal sinus, dura, falx cerebri, tentorium and brain with distinct white and grey matter, as shown in Fig. 1.5. This head was developed to incorporate the Total Human Model for Safety (THUMS), a FE model of the entire human body. The model was validated for head-neck motions, lateral bending and rear end impact (Iwamoto 2003) and for experiments on cadavers (Hardy et al. 2001; Nahum et al. 1977; Trosseille et al. 1992). THUMS was also tested with SUFHEM, showing comparable results (Ipek et al. 2009).

More recently, Mao et al. (2013) developed a new FEHM with precise geometries and validated it for several experimental cases. This head model was integrated into the full body model supported by the Global Human Body Models Consortium (GHBMC) (Schwartz et al. 2015). This model is composed by scalp, skull, meninges, bridging veins and brain with distinct white and grey matter. Only the meninges were modelled as linear elastic. The others were modelled as viscoelastic or elastic-plastic materials. This model was validated by Mao et al. (2013) for a huge number of experimental tests, such as brain pressure (Nahum et al. 1977; Trosseille et al. 1992),

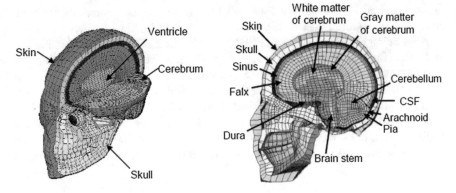

Fig. 1.5 THUMS model (adopted from Iwamoto et al. 2007)

brain motion (Hardy et al. 2001), skull response (Hodgson et al. 1970; Yoganandan et al. 1995), among others. Nevertheless, significant discrepancies between simulated and experimental results were observed in a great number of different tests.

More information about these and other models can be found in Raul et al. (2008) and Tse et al. (2014). At the point this work is written, models such as SUFEHM, WSUHIM, KTH, UCDBTM and GHBMC represent the cutting-edge state-of-art for FEHM. All of these use nonlinear material models to simulate brain's behaviour. Although a great number of FEHMs exist, gyri and sulci are absent in almost all these models. In these, brain's global geometry is usually similar to a ellipsoidal structure without sulci and gyri. Basically, a simplified volume resembling a brain with a smooth surface.

Cloots et al. (2008) reported that gyri and sulci had a significant effect on maximum von Mises stress value. Cloots et al. (2010) indicated that a well-defined correlation between mechanical loading and DAI using FEHM has not been achieved yet. A possible contribution to this is absence of gyri and sulci in brain models, which can play an important role in the local tissue deformations (Cloots et al. 2008; Lauret et al. 2009). The folding structure of the brain surface and the non-uniform distribution of the CSF greatly influence both the distribution and the magnitude of the maximum stress and strains in the brain (Cloots et al. 2008; Gilchrist and O'Donoghue 2000; Lauret et al. 2009). In addition, Ho and Kleiven (2009) verified that strain and strain rates during impacts were both reduced in a model with sulci (Ho et al. 2009), especially for rotational accelerations in the sagittal plane. They also concluded that the presence of these structures should be considered in future models.

In addition, the relative motion between skull and brain is also important. The majority of these models have different components with shared or rigidly connected nodes, which influence the brain's intracranial motion. Little attention has been paid to the relative motion between structures. Excessive motion between skull and brain may injure brain's surface or even the bridging veins connecting them, which may rupture under excessive loading (Horgan and Gilchrist 2003; Tse et al. 2014). This may cause damage on the brain's surface (sulci and gyri) and even in the brain tissue. Cerebral contusions usually involve the surface of the brain, especially the crowns of gyri (Gurdjian et al. 1966; Ommaya et al. 1971).

After being properly validated, FEHMs can be used as an injury evaluation tool in accident reconstructions and forensic cases (Tchepel et al. 2016b), in testing new materials and technologies for safety applications (Fernandes et al. 2015, 2017a, b; Ptak et al. 2017a) and even in the design and optimisation of personal safety gear such as helmets (Fernandes and Alves de Sousa 2013; Fernandes et al. 2013; Ptak et al. 2017b). In the following chapters, it is described the development of a new FEHM with a brain model with sulci and gyri that also allows the brain to move inside the skull. This model is a new contribution to the state-of-the-art of FEHMs.

References

N. Andaluz, Traumatic brain injury. Mayfield Clinic (2016)

M. Aare, Prevention of head injuries focusing specifically on oblique impacts. Doctoral thesis, Technical Report 2003-26, School of Technology and Health, Royal Institute of Technology, Stockholm, Sweden, 2003

M. Aare, S. Kleiven, P. Halldin, Injury criteria for oblique helmet impacts, in *Proceedings of IRCOBI Conference*, Lisbon (Portugal) (2003), pp. 349–350

S.H. Advani, W. Powell, J. Huston, S.J. Ojala, Human head impact response—experimental data and analytical simulations, in *Proceedings of IRCOBI*, Birmingham (1975), pp. 153–163

S. Advani, A. Ommaya, W. Yang, Head injury mechanisms, in *Human Body Dynamics*, ed. by D.N. Ghista (Oxford University Press, 1982)

M. Aiello, U. Galvanetto, L. Iannucci, Numerical simulations of motorcycle helmet impact tests. Int. J. Crashworthiness **12**, 1–7 (2007)

A.S. Al-Bsharat, W.N. Hardy, K.H. Yang, T.B. Khalil, S. Tashman, A.I. King, Brain/skull relative displacement magnitude due to blunt head imapact: new experimental data and model, in *Proceedings of the 43rd Stapp Car Crash Conference* (1999), pp. 321–332, Paper No. 99SC22

D. Allsop, C. Warner, M. Wille, D. Schneider, A. Nahum, Facial impact response—a comparison of the Hybrid III dummy and the human cadaver, in *Proceeding of 32nd Stapp Car Crash Conference, SAE 881719*, Atlanta (1988)

D. Allsop, T. Perl, C. Warner, Force/deflection and fracture characteristics of the temporo-parietal of the human head, in *Proceedings of 35th Stapp Car Crash Conference, SAE 912907*, San Diego (1991), pp. 139–155

R. Anderson, A study of the biomechanics of axonal injury. Ph.D. thesis, University of Adelaide, 2000

B.C. Bain, D.F. Meaney, Tissue-level thresholds for axonal damage in an experimental model of central nervous system white matter injury. J. Biomech. Eng. **122**(6), 615–622 (2000)

F.A. Bandak, On the mechanics of impact neurotrauma: a review and critical synthesis. J. Neurotrauma **12**(4), 635–649 (1995)

F.A. Bandak, Biomechanics of impact traumatic brain injury, in *Crashworthiness of Transportation Systems: Structural Impact and Occupant Protection*, ed. by J.A.C. Ambrosio, M.F.O. Seabra Pereira, P.F. Silva (Springer Netherlands, Dordrecht, 1997a), pp. 53–93

F.A. Bandak, Impact traumatic brain injury: a mechanical perspective, in *Neurotraumatology-Biomechanic Aspects, Cytologic and Molecular Mechanisms*, ed. by M. Oehmichen, H.G. König (Lübeck, Schmidt-Römhild, 1997b), pp. 59–83

F.A. Bandak, R.H Eppinger, A three-dimensional FE analysis of the human brain under combined rotational and translational accelerations, in *Proceedings of 38th Stapp Car Crash Conference, Society of Automotive Engineers* (1994), pp. 145–163

F.A. Bandak, A.X. Zhang, R.E. Tannous, F. DiMasi, P. Masiello, R. Eppinger, SIMon: a simulated injury monitor: application to head injury assessment, in *Proceedings of the 17th International Technical Conference on the Enhanced Safety of Vehicles (ESV)*, Amsterdam, The Netherlands (2001)

D. Baumgartner, Mécanismes de lésion et limites de tolérance au choc de la tête humaine-Reconstruction numérique et expérimentale de traumatismes créniens. Ph.D. Dissertation, Université Louis Pasteur Strasbourg, 2001

D. Baumgartner, R. Willinger, N. Shewchenko, M. Beusenberg, Tolerance limits for mild traumatic brain injury derived from numerical head impact replication, in *Proceedings of IRCOBI Conference*, Isle of Man, UK (2001)

G. Belingardi, G. Chiandussi, I. Gaviglio, *Development and Validation of a New Finite Element Model of Human Head*, Politecnico di Torino, Dipartimento di Meccanica, Italy, Paper Number 05-0441 (2005)

D.W. Brands, P.H. Bovendeerd, J.S.H.M. Wismans, On the potential importance of non-linear viscoelastic material modelling for numerical prediction of brain tissue response, in *Proceedings 46th Stapp Car Crash Conference*, SAE paper vol 2002-22-0006 (2002), pp. 103–121

B. Canaple, G. Rungen, E. Markiewicz, P. Drazetic, J. Happian-Smith, B. Chinn, D. Cesari, Impact model development for the reconstruction of current motorcycle accidents. Int. J. Crashworthiness **7**(3), 307–320 (2002)

B. Canaple, G. Rungen, P. Drazetic, E. Markiewicz, D. Cesari, Towards a finite element head model used as a head injury predictive tool. Int. J. Crashworthiness **8**(1), 41–52 (2003)

L. Cardamone. Analisi numerica del trauma cranico da impatto. Technical Report (Bioengineering Laboratory, University of Salerno, Italy, 2005)

M.S. Chafi, G. Karami, M. Ziejewski, Biomechanical assessment of brain dynamic responses due to blast pressure waves. Ann. Biomed. Eng. **38**(2), 490–504 (2009)

M. Claessens, F. Sauren, J. Wismans, Modeling of the human head under impact conditions: a parametric study. SAE Transactions Paper No. 973338 (1997), pp. 3829–3848

R.J.H. Cloots, H.M.T. Gervaise, J.A.W. van Dommelen, M.G.D. Geers, Biomechanics of traumatic brain injury: influences of the morphologic heterogeneities of the cerebral cortex. Ann. Biomed. Eng. **36**(7), 1203–1215 (2008)

R.J.H. Cloots, J.A.W. van Dommelen, S. Kleiven, M.G.D. Geers, Traumatic brain injury at multiple length scales: relating diffuse axonal injury to discrete axonal impairment, in *Proceedings of IRCOBI Conference*, Hanover, Germany (2010), pp .119–130

COST327, (2001) Motorcycle safety helmets. Final report of the action, European Communities, Belgium

K.K. Darvish, J.R. Crandall, Influence of brain material properties and boundary conditions on brain response during dynamic loading, in *Proceedings of IRCOBI Conference*, Munich, Germany (2002)

C. Deck, R. Willinger, Improved head injury criteria based on head FE model. Int. J. Crashworthiness **13**(6), 667–679 (2008)

C. Deck, R. Willinger, Head injury prediction tool for predictive systems optimization, in *Proceedings of 7th European LS-DYNA Conference* (2009)

C. Deck, B. Baumgartner, R. Willinger, Helmet optimisation on head-helmet modelling. Struct. Mater. **13**, 319–328 (2003)

F. DiMasi, J. Marcus, R. Eppinger, Three dimensional anatomic brain model for relating cortical strains to automobile crash loading, in *Proceedings of the 12th International Technical Conference on Experimental Safety Vehicles, NHTSA*, Washington, vol. 2 (1991), pp. 617–627

F. DiMasi, R.H. Eppinger, F.A. Bandak, Computational analysis of head impact response under car crash loadings, in *Proceedings of 39th Stapp Car Crash Conference, Society of Automotive Engineers, SAE Paper No. 952718, Society of Automotive Engineers*, Warrendale, PA (1995), pp. 425–438

V. Dirisala, G. Karami, M. Ziejewski, Effects of neck damping properties on brain response under impact loading. Int. J. Numer. Methods Biomed. Eng. **28**(4), 472–494 (2011)

Y. Dokko, R.W.G. Anderson, J. Manavis, P.C. Blumbergs, A.J. McLean, L. Zhang, K.H. Yang, A.I. King, Validation of the human head FE model against pedestrian accidents and its tentative application to the examination of the existing tolerance curve, in *Proceedings of 18th International Technical Conference on the Enhanced Safety of Vehicles*, ESV, Nagoya, Japan (2003)

M.C. Doorly, M.D. Gilchrist, The use of accident reconstruction for the analysis of traumatic brain injury due to head impacts arising from falls. Comput. Methods Biomech. Biomed. Eng. **9**(6), 371–377 (2006)

F.A.O. Fernandes, R.J. Alves de Sousa, Finite element analysis of helmeted oblique impacts and head injury evaluation with a commercial road helmet. Struct. Eng. Mech. **48**(5), 661–679 (2013)

F.A.O. Fernandes, R.J. Alves de Sousa, Head injury predictors in sports trauma—A state-of-the-art review. Proc. Inst. Mech. Eng. Part H: J. Eng. Med. **229**(8), 592–608 (2015)

F.A.O. Fernandes, R.J. Alves de Sousa, W. Willinger, C. Deck, Finite element analysis of helmeted impacts and head injury evaluation with a commercial road helmet, in *IRCOBI Conference Proceedings—International Research Council on the Biomechanics of Injury*, Gothenburg, Sweden (2013), pp. 431–442, September

F.A.O. Fernandes, R.T. Jardin, A.B. Pereira, R.J. Alves de Sousa, Comparing the mechanical performance of synthetic and natural cellular materials. Mater. Des. **82**, 335–341 (2015)

F.A.O. Fernandes, J.P. Tavares, R.J. Alves de Sousa, A.B. Pereira, J.P. Esteves, Manufacturing and testing composites based on natural materials. Procedia Manuf. **13**, 227–234 (2017a)

F.A.O. Fernandes, D.F. Oliveira, A.B. Pereira, Optimal parameters for laser welding of advanced high-strength steels used in the automotive industry. Procedia Manuf. **13**, 219–226 (2017b)

M. Franklyn, B. Fildes, R. Dwarampudi, L. Zhang, K. Yang, L. Sparke, R. Eppinger, Analysis of computer models for head injury investigation, in *Proceedings of the 18th International Technical Conference on Enhanced Safety Vehicles* (2003)

M.D. Gilchrist, D. O'Donoghue, Simulation of the development of frontal head impact injury. Comput. Mech. **26**, 229–235 (2000)

C. Giordano, R.J.H. Cloots, J.A.W. van Dommelen, S. Kleiven, The influence of anisotropy on brain injury prediction. J. Biomech. **47**, 1052–1059 (2014)

E.S. Gurdjian, H.R. Lissner, V.R. Hodgson et al., Mechanisms of head injury. Clin. Neurosurg. **12**, 112–128 (1966)

W.N. Hardy, C.D. Foster, M.J. Mason, K.H. King, A.I. King, S. Tashman, Investigation of head injury mechanisms using neutral density technology and high-speed biplanar X-ray. Stapp Car Crash J. **45**, 337–368 (2001)

U. Hartmann, F. Kruggel, Trasient analysis of the biomechanics of the human head with a high-resolution 3D finite element model. Comput. Methods Biomech. Biomed. Eng. **2**(1), 49–64 (1999)

J. Ho, S. Kleiven, Dynamic response of the brain with vasculature: a three-dimensional computational study. J. Biomech. **40**, 3006–3012 (2007)

J. Ho, S. Kleiven, Can sulci protect the brain from traumatic injury? J. Biomech. **42**, 2074–2080 (2009)

J. Ho, H. von Holst, S. Kleiven, Automatic generation and validation of patient-specific finite element head models suitable for crashworthiness analysis. Int. J. Crashworthiness **14**(6), 555–563 (2009)

V.R. Hodgson, L.M. Thomas, Breaking strength of the human skull versus impact surface curvature. Report, Department of Neurosurgery, Wayne State University School of Medicine (1971)

Hodgson, V R., Brinn, J., Thomas, L.M., Greenberg, S.W., 1970. Fracture Behavior of the Skull Frontal Bone Against Cylindrical Surfaces. Proceedings of 14th Stapp Car Crash Conference, SAE International, Warrendale, PA

T.J. Horgan, M.D. Gilchrist, The creation of three-dimensional finite element models for simulating head impact biomechanics. Int. J. Crashworthiness **8**(4), 353–366 (2003)

T.J. Horgan, M.D. Gilchrist, Influence of FE model variability in predicting brain motion and intracranial pressure changes in head impact simulations. Int. J. Crashworthiness **9**(4), 401–418 (2004)

R.R. Hosey, Y.K. Liu, A homeomorphic finite element model of the human head and neck, in *Finite Elements in Biomechanics, chapter 18*, ed. by B.R. Simon, R.H. Gallagher, P.C. Johnson, J.F. Gross (Wiley, France, 1982), pp. 379–401

M. Hrapko, J.A.W. van Dommelen, G.W.M. Peters, J.S.H.M. Wismans, The influence of test conditions on characterization of the mechanical properties of brain tissue. J. Biomech. Eng. **130**(3), 663–676 (2008)

A. Hume, N.J. Mills, A. Gilchrist, Industrial head injuries and the performance of the helmets, in *Proceedings of IRCOBI Conference*, Brunnen, Switzerland (1995), pp. 217–231

H. Ipek, C. Mayer, C. Deck, H. Luce, P. de Gueselle, R. Willinger, Coupling of Strasbourg University head model to thums human body FE model: validation and application to automotive safety. Paper number 09–0384 (2009), pp. 1–13

M. Iwamoto, Recent Advances in THUMS: development of the detailed head-neck and internal organs, and THUMS family. *LS-DYNA & JMAG User Conference*, Japan (2003)

M. Iwamoto, K. Yoshikatsu, I. Watanabe, K. Furusu, K. Miki, J. Hasegawa, Development of a finite element model of the total human model for safety (thums) and application to injury reconstruction, in *Proceedings of IRCOBI Conference*, Munich, Germany (2002)

M. Iwamoto, Y. Nakahira, A. Tamura, H. Kimpara, I. Watanabe, K. Miki, Development of advanced human models in thums. *6th European LS-DYNA Users Conference* (2007), pp. 47–56

H. Kang, R. Willinger, B.M. Diaw, B. Chinn, Validation of a 3D anatomic human head model and replication of head impact in motorcycle accident by finite element modelling. SAE Transactions Paper No. 973339 (1997), pp. 849–858

T.B. Khalil, R.P. Hubbard, Parametric study of head response by finite element modelling. J. Biomech. **10**, 119–132 (1977)

T.B. Khalil, D.C. Viano, Critical issues in finite element modelling of head impact, in *Proceedings of 26th Stapp Car Crash Conference, SAE paper*, vol. 821150 (1982), pp. 87–102

J.E. Kim, Y.H. Kim, Z. Li, A.W. Eberhardt, B.K. Soni, Evaluation of traumatic brain injury using multi-body and finite element models, in *17th IMACS World Congress, Scientific Computation, Applied Mathematics and Simulation*, Paris, France (2005)

H. Kimpara, Y. Nakahira, M. Iwamoto, K. Miki, K. Ichihara, T. Kawano Taguchi, Investigation of anteroposterior head-neck responses during severe frontal impacts using a brain-spinal cord complex FE model, in *Proceedings 50th Stapp Car Crash Conference* (2006), pp. 509–544

A. King, K. Yang, L. Zhang, W. Hardy, D. Viano, Is head injury caused by linear or angular acceleration? in *Proceedings of IRCOBI Conference*, Lisbon (2003), pp. 1–10

S. Kleiven, Finite element modeling of the human head. Doctoral thesis, Technical Report, School of Technology an Health, Royal Institute of Technology, Stockholm, Sweden, 2002

S. Kleiven, Biomechanics as a forensic science tool—Reconstruction of a traumatic head injury using the finite element method. Scand. J. Forensic Sci. **2**, 73–78 (2006a)

S. Kleiven, Evaluation of head injury criteria using an FE model validated against experiments on localized brain motion, intra-cerebral acceleration, and intra-cranial pressure. Int. J. Crashworthiness **11**(1), 65–79 (2006b)

S. Kleiven, *Head Injury Biomechanics and Criteria. Biomechanics and Neuronics*, course literature, KTH (2007a)

S. Kleiven, Predictors for traumatic brain injuries evaluated through accident reconstructions, in *Proceedings of the 51st Stapp Car Crash Conference* (2007b), pp. 81–114

S. Kleiven, W.N. Hardy, Correlation of an FE model of the human head with experiments on localized motion of the brain: consequences for injury prediction, in Proceedings 45th Stapp Car Crash J. Society of Automotive Engineers, SAE Paper No. 02S-76 (2002)

S. Kleiven, H. von Holst, Consequences of brain size following impact in prediction of subdural hematoma evaluated with numerical techniques, in *Proceedings of IRCOBI Conference*, Isle of Man, UK (2001), pp. 161–172

S. Kleiven, H. von Holst, Consequences of head size following trauma to the human head. J. Biomech. **35**(2), 153–160 (2002)

G. Krabbel, R. Müller, Development of a finite element model of the head using the visible human data, in *Abstracts of the Visible Human Project Conference*, Bethesda (1996), pp. 71–72

C. Lauret, M. Hrapko, J.A.W. van Dommelen, G.W.M. Peters, J.S.H.M. Wismans, Optical characterization of acceleration-induced strain fields in inhomogeneous brain slices. Med. Eng. Phys. **31**, 392–399 (2009)

M.C. Lee, R.C. Haut, Insensitivity of tensile failure properties of human bridging veins to strain rate: Implications in biomechanics of subdural hematoma. J. Biomech. **22**, 537–542 (1989)

X. Li, H. von Holst, S. Kleiven, Influence of gravity for optimal head positions in the treatment of head injury patients. Acta Neurochir. **153**, 2057–2064 (2011)

D.S. Liu, C.M. Fan, Applied pressure tolerance to evaluate motorcycle helmet design, in *Proceedings of International Crashworthiness Conference*, Dearborn, Michigan, USA (1998)

P. Löwenhielm, Strain tolerance of the Vv. Cerebri Sup. (bridging veins) calculated from head-on collision tests with cadavers. Z. fur Rechtsmed. **75**(2), 131–144 (1974)

H. Mao, L. Zhang, B. Jiang et al., Development of a finite element human head model partially validated with thirty five experimental cases. J. Biomech. Eng. **135**, 111002–15 (2013)

S.S. Margulies, L.E. Thibault, A proposed tolerance criterion for diffuse axonal injury in man. J. Biomech. **25**(8), 917–923 (1992)

D. Marjoux, D. Baumgartner, C. Deck, R. Willinger, Head injury prediction capability of the HIC, HIP, SIMon and ULP criteria. Accid. Anal. Prev. **40**(3), 1135–1148 (2008)

T.W. McAllister, J.C. Ford, S. Ji, J.G. Beckwith, L.A. Flashman, K. Paulsen, R.M. Greenwald, Maximum principal strain and strain rate associated with concussion diagnosis correlates with changes in corpus callosum white matter indices. Ann. Biomed. Eng. **40**(1), 127–140 (2012)

J.H. McElhaney, J.H. Fogle, J.W. Melvin, R.R. Haynes, V.L. Roberts, N.B. Alem, Mechanical properties of cranial bone. J. Biomech. **3**, 495–511 (1970)

A. McKinlay, A. Bishop, T. McLellan, Public knowledge of "concussion" and the different terminology used to communicate about mild traumatic brain injury. Brain Inj. **25**, 761–766 (2011)

A.J. McLean, Brain injury without head impact? J. Neurotrauma **12**, 621–625 (1995)

J.W. Melvin, J.H. McElhaney, V.L. Roberts, Development of a mechanical model of the human head—determination of tissue properties and synthetic substitute materials, in *Proceedings of 14th Stapp Car Crash Conference, Society of Automotive Engineers*, SAE Paper No. 700903 (1970)

K. Mendis, Finite element modelling of the brain to establish diffuse axonal injury criteria. Ph.D. Dissertation, Ohio State University, 1992

R.T. Miller, S.S. Margulies, M. Leoni, M. Nonaka, X.H. Chen, D.H. Smith, D.F. Meaney, Finite element modeling approaches for predicting injury in an experimental model of severe diffuse axonal injury, in *Proceedings of 42nd Stapp Car Crash Conference*, SAE Paper 983154 (1998), pp. 155–166

A.G. Monea, G. Van der Perre, K. Baeck, H. Delye, P. Verschueren, E. Forauseberzher, C. Van Lierdem, I. Verpoestm, J.V. Slotenm, J. Goffin, B. Depreitere, The relation between mechanical impact parameters and most frequent bicycle related head injuries. J. Mech. Behav. Biomed. Mater. **33**, 3–15 (2014)

K.L. Monson, W. Goldsmith, N.M. Barbaro, G.T. Manley, Axial mechanical properties of fresh human cerebral blood vessels. J. Biomech. Eng. **125**(2), 288–294 (2003)

B. Morrison III, H.L. Cater, C.C.B. Wang, F.C. Thomas, C.T. Hung, G.A. Ateshian, L.E. Sundström, A tissue level tolerance criterion for living brain developed in an in vitro model of traumatic mechanical loading, in *Proceedings of 47th Stapp Car Crash Conference*, SAE Paper No. 2003-22-0006 (2003)

J. Motherway, M.C. Doorly, M. Curtis, M.D. Gilchrist, Head impact biomechanics simulations: a forensic tool for reconstructing head injury? Leg. Med. **11**, S220–S222 (2009)

A. Nahum, J. Gatts, C. Gadd, J. Danforth, Impact tolerance of the skull and face, in *Proceedings of 12nd Stapp Car Crash Conference*, SAE 680785, Detroit (1968)

A.M. Nahum, R. Smith, C.C. Ward, Intracranial pressure dynamics during head impact, in *Proceeding of 21st Stapp Car Crash Conference* (1977), pp. 339–366

R. Willinger, H.S. Kang, B.M. Diaw, Développement et validation d'un modéle mècanique de la tête humaine (Development and validation of a human head mechanical model). Comptes Rendus de l'Académie des Sciences-Series IIB-Mechanics-Physics-Astronomy **327**(1), 125–131 (1999a)

R. Willinger, H.S. Kang, B.M. Diaw, Three-dimensional human head finite-element model validation against two experimental impacts. Ann. Biomed. Eng. **27**(3), 403–410 (1999b)

R. Willinger, D. Baumgartner, B. Chinn, M. Neale, Head tolerance limits derived from numerical replication of real world accidents, in *Proceedings of IRCOBI Conference*, Isle of Man, UK (2000a), pp. 209–222

R. Willinger, D. Baumgartner, T. Guimberteau, Dynamic characterization of motorcycle helmets: modelling and coupling with the human head. J. Sound Vib. **235**, 611–625 (2000b)

R. Willinger, B.M. Diaw, H.S. Kang, Finite element modeling of skull fractures caused by direct impact. Int. J. Crashworthiness **5**(3), 249–258 (2000c)

R.M. Wright, K.T. Ramesh, An axonal strain injury criterion for traumatic brain injury. Biomech. Model. Mechanobiol. **11**, 245–260 (2012)

W. Yan, O.D. Pangestu, A modified human head model for the study of impact head injury. Comput. Methods Biomech. Biomed. Eng. **14**(12), 1049–1057 (2011)

J. Yang, Investigation of brain trauma biomechanics in vehicle traffic accidents using human body computational models, in *Computational Biomechanics for Medicine: Soft Tissues and the Musculoskeletal System*, ed. by A. Wittek et al. (Springer Science+Business Media LLC, 2011)

J. Yao, J. Yang, J. Otte, Investigation of brain injuries by reconstructions of real world adult pedestrian accidents, in *Proceedings of IRCOBI Conference*, Madrid, Spain (2006), pp. 241–252

J.F. Yao, J.K. Yang, D. Otte, Investigation of head injuries by reconstructions of real-world vehicle-versus-adult-pedestrian accidents. Saf. Sci. **46**(7), 1103–1114 (2008)

N. Yoganandan, A. Sances, F.A. Pintar, P.R. Walsh, C.L. Ewing, D.J. Thomas, R.G. Snyder, J. Reinartz, K. Droese, Biomechanical tolerance of the cranium. SAE Transactions Paper No. 94172, Warrendale (1994), pp. 184–188

N. Yoganandan, F.A. Pintar, A. Sances, E.R. Walsh, C.L. Ewing, D.J. Thomas, R.G. Snyder, Biomechanics of skull fracture. J. Neurotrauma **12**(4), 659–668 (1995)

L. Zhang, K. Yang, R. Dwarampudi, K. Omori, T. Li, K. Chang, W.N. Hardy, T.B. Khalil, A.I. King, Recent advances in brain injury research: a new human head model development and validation. Stapp Car Crash J. **45**, 369–394 (2001)

L. Zhang, K.H. Yang, A.I. King, D.C. Viano, A new biomechanical predictor for mild traumatic brain injury—a preliminary finding, in *ASME Bioengineering Conference Proceedings*, Florida, USA (2003), pp. 25–29

L. Zhang, K. Yang, A. King, A proposed injury threshold for mild traumatic brain injury. J. Biomech. Eng. **126**(2), 226–236 (2004)

J. Zhang, N. Yoganandan, F.A. Pintar, Y. Guan, T.A. Gennarelli, *Biomechanical Differences Between Contact and Non-contact Head Impacts in Vehicle Crash Tests*. Department of Neurosurgery, Medical College of Wisconsin, United States, Paper Number 07-0352 (2007)

L. Zhang, K. Yang, T.A. Gennarelli, Mathematical modeling of cerebral concussion: correlations of regional brain strain with clinical symptoms, in *Proceedings of IRCOBI Conference*, Bern, Switzerland (2008), pp. 123–132

C. Zhou, T.B. Khalil, A.I. King, A new model comparing impact responses of the homogeneous and inhomogeneous human brain, in *Proceedings of 39th Stapp Car Crash Conference, Society of Automotive Engineers* (1995), pp. 121–137

C. Zhou, T.B. Kahlil, L.J. Dragovic, Head injury assessment of a real world crash by finite element modelling, in *Proceedings of the Advisory Group for Aerospace Research and Development, AGARD-Conference Proceedings*, New Mexico (1996), pp. 81–87

M. Ziejewski, G. Karami, W.W. Orrison, E.H. Hanson, Dynamic response of head under vehicle crash loading. Paper 09-0432, in *Proceedings of the 21st International Conference on the Enhanced Safety of Vehicles (ESV)*, NHTSA, Washington DC (2009)

Chapter 2
Development of a New Finite Element Human Head Model

2.1 Introduction

Traumatic brain injury (TBI) is one of the main causes of death and disability. TBI occurs when a load exceeds the brain tissue tolerance level (Fernandes and Alves de Sousa 2015). Road traffic accidents, sports, assaults and work and home accidents are the major sources. In some of these, the evolution of protective head gear is extremely important. One way of biomechanically optimising head protective devices is by using a FEHM.

Once properly validated, a FEHM can be used in protective gear design and in the reconstruction of injurious events, by predicting brain injuries under several impact conditions. Finite element analysis (FEA) allows to compute variables such as stress and strain, which would be infeasible experimentally (measuring in-vivo). Variables such as strain have been pointed out as better injury indicators than externally measured linear or angular acceleration. Due to legal and ethical reasons as well as the risk of injury, obtaining data from living human subjects is impossible. In the late 1970s, Nahum et al. (1977) performed impact experiments on cadavers. Currently, the results from this publication are still being used as reference in FEHM's validation.

In order to better understand the mechanisms of TBI, several research groups have developed FEHMs, some of them with detailed geometric descriptions of anatomical features and different material properties (Horgan and Gilchrist 2003; Kleiven 2007b; Ruan and Prasad 1995; Sahoo et al. 2014a; Takhounts et al. 2008; Yang 2011; Zhang et al. 2011). Detailed information about these models and the evolution of FEHMs is presented in Sect. 1.2.

The first FEHMs appeared between the late 1970s and early 1980s. These were simple 2D models with some questionable results. Since then, the biomechanics of the brain for injury analysis and prevention has been a very active area of research (Miller 2011). With the increasing CPU power, more complex models have been developed.

More realistic 3D models were only possible in the 90s and further with the advances in computing (Horgan and Gilchrist 2003; Kleiven 2007b; Mao et al. 2013; Sahoo et al. 2014a; Takhounts et al. 2008; Yang 2011; Zhang et al. 2001). These are

© The Author(s) 2018
F. A. O. Fernandes et al., *Head Injury Simulation in Road Traffic Accidents*, SpringerBriefs in Applied Sciences and Technology, https://doi.org/10.1007/978-3-319-89926-8_2

the more complex ones found in the literature. There are a great number of other models, but these are oversimplified or not validated.

Although a great number of FEHMs exist, gyri and sulci are absent in almost all these models. In these, brain's global geometry is usually similar to spheroidal/ellipsoidal structures, without sulci and gyri. Basically, a simplified volume resembling a brain with a smooth surface. Cloots et al. (2008), using a 2D FE model, reported that gyri and sulci had a significant effect on von Mises stress maximum value. Additionally, Cloots et al. (2010) indicated that a well-defined correlation between mechanical loading and DAI using FEHM has not been achieved yet. A possible contribution to this is absence of gyri and sulci in brain models, which can play an important role in the local tissue deformations (Cloots et al. 2008; Lauret et al. 2009). The folding structure of the brain surface and the non-uniform distribution of the CSF greatly influence both the distribution and the magnitude of the maximum stress and strains in the brain (Cloots et al. 2008; Gilchrist and O'Donoghue 2000; Lauret et al. 2009). In addition, Ho and Kleiven (2009) verified that strain and strain rates during impacts were both reduced in a model with sulci, especially for rotational accelerations in the sagittal plane. They also concluded that the presence of these structures should be considered in future models. Figure 2.1 shows in detail sulci and gyri structures.

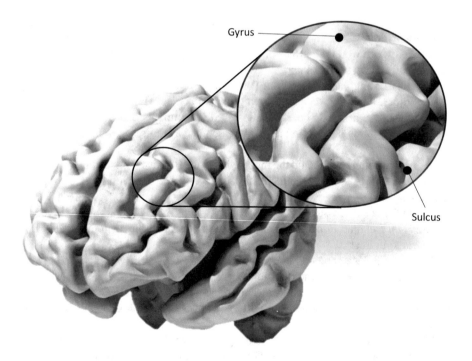

Fig. 2.1 Illustration of the structures gyri and sulci

The relative motion between skull and brain is also important to model. The majority of these models have shared or rigidly connected nodes, which influence the brain's intracranial motion. Little attention has been paid to the relative motion between structures. Supported on this, Claessens et al. (1997) created a geometrically simple FEHM where structures inside the head have the ability to move relative to one another.

Excessive relative motion between skull and brain may injure brain's surface or even the bridging veins connecting them, which may rupture under excessive loading (Horgan and Gilchrist 2003; Tse et al. 2014). In addition, excessive relative motion may cause damage on the brain's surface (sulci and gyri) and even inside the brain. Cerebral contusions usually involve the surface of the brain, especially the crowns of gyri (Gurdjian et al. 1966; Ommaya et al. 1971).

Thus, in this chapter, it is presented the modelling and validation of a FEHM with a brain model with sulci and gyri. This model will also allow the brain to move inside the skull. The model developed and validated in this work can give a great contribution in predicting brain injuries, using also proper criteria. For instance, cerebral contusions due to the geometrical detail of the brain surface.

2.2 Methods and Materials

In this work, a FEHM is developed. Different steps were necessary to model it: geometric modelling, material modelling, contact definition and validation. In order to validate it, the experiments performed by Nahum et al. (1977) and Hardy et al. (2001) in cadavers were simulated. These are important to validate the brain response in terms of pressure and motion, respectively.

2.2.1 Geometric Modelling

In this work, the head modelled is based on medical images. These are typically used to correctly model the human body. Computer tomography (CT) and magnetic resonance imaging (MRI) are usually used to observe what is happening inside our bodies. The first technique, CT, is normally employed to observe bone structures, whereas MRI technique is suitable for soft tissues. Thus, in this work, CT and MRI were used to generate the skull's and brain's geometry, respectively.

In order to accurately generate skull's geometry, 460 images spaced 1.5 mm and obtained from CT scans were used. From this set of slices, the skull's geometry was extracted by creating a region of interest (ROI) with the Osirix software (Osirix 2003). This skull's ROI was created by automatic segmentation using Osirix's plug-in, MIA. Afterwards, this ROI was manually adjusted in some slices at the sagittal and coronal planes in order to improve the skull's geometry, as shown in Fig. 2.2.

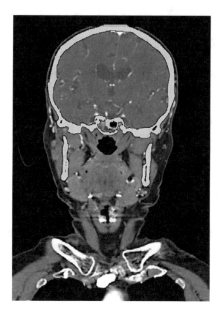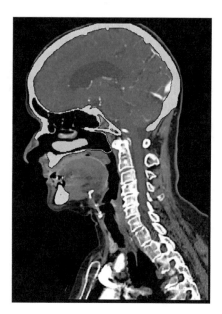

Fig. 2.2 CT scans used to model the skull geometry

Brain's geometry was generated from segmentation of MRI data, employing the same technique used for the skull. The MRI data consisted of 181 T2-weighted slices taken at 1 mm intervals in a human male head. With T2 weighted images, it was possible to distinguish the brain from the other intracranial contents. Some manual adjustments were applied at all the three planes, sagittal, coronal and axial, in order to improve the skull's geometry. Nevertheless, after manual segmentation and geometry generation, some irregularities and deviations were still present. These were lightly smoothed using Meshmixer software (Meshmixer 2012), without compromising the model's global geometry. In addition, a software named Meshlab was also used in order to close any existing gaps in the triangular mesh of the geometric model (STereoLithography (STL) model) (Cignoni et al. 2008). Both STL meshes have a suitable amount of triangles, generating precise geometries without overloading the computer.

These STL models were then imported to CATIA V5 in order to create 3D solid computer-aided design (CAD) models (CATIA V5 2008). After successfully generating skull and brain CAD models, the space between skull and brain was used to model the CSF. In other words, brain and skull models acted as "sculpting moulds" in the modelling of CSF, as shown in Fig. 2.3. Finally, these CAD models were imported into Abaqus, creating the FE meshes. Figure 2.3 shows a summary of the methodology used to create the geometry of the YEt Another Head Model (YEAHM).

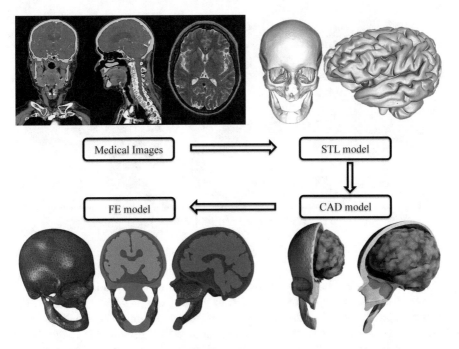

Fig. 2.3 Methodology used to model YEAHM geometry

2.2.2 Description of the YEAHM

The human brain can be simply described as a soft highly metabolically active tissue, floating in CSF within the rigid cranium (Bilston 2011). These protect the brain from external mechanical loads experienced by the head during normal daily life. Thus, YEAHM consists of skull, CSF and brain as shown in Fig. 2.4. This shows a cross section of the model and illustrates the anatomical features of the head.

The brain model has all important sections: frontal, parietal, temporal, and occipital lobes, both hemispheres, cerebrum, cerebellum, corpus callosum, thalamus, midbrain, and brain stem. It was not possible to separately segment CSF and structures such as membranes and bridging veins because of the resolution of MRI data. Then, a volume was created to represent all these parts between skull and brain. It was named as CSF due to its larger volume. Also, there is no consensus if cerebral vasculature should be included or not in head modelling (Ho and Kleiven 2007; Zhang et al. 2002).

In addition, the cerebral ventricular system was also modelled and filled with CSF. The CSF is described using solid elements with a low shear modulus, as in other publications (Yang 2011). The global CSF model is a combination of the CSF and the meninges. For instance, the inner surface of the CSF model acts as the pia mater, surrounding the brain and dipping down into sulci and fissures and thus, acquiring the brain shape.

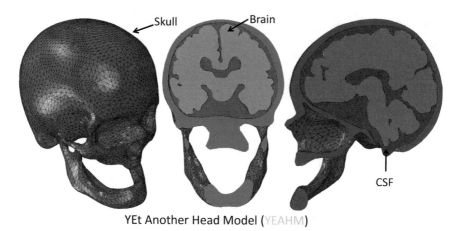

YEt Another Head Model (YEAHM)

Fig. 2.4 YEAHM consists of skull (blue), CSF (red) and brain (green)

The adult human skull is made up of eight bones that are rigidly connected by sutures. For this reason, there is no need to model them as separate bones. It has been reported that the skull thickness can vary from 4 to 9 mm (Kleiven 2002; Ruan and Prasad 2001). YEAHM's skull has a variable thickness in this range, being geometrically accurate. In addition, most FEHMs developed so far have a skull with uniform thickness (Yang and King 2011).

In addition to the ventricles and the skull with a variable thickness, the latter was also modelled with some of its real irregularities at the base. Ivarsson et al. (2002) indicated that the ventricles and the irregular skull base are necessary in modelling head impact, since the latter protects nerves and vessels passing through the cranial floor by reducing brain displacement. Ivarsson et al. (2002) also concluded that CSF relieves strain in regions inferior and superior to the ventricles. This is supported by Kleiven (2005), observing also low levels of strain in the vicinity of the ventricles, probably due to strain relief around them.

All parts were modelled as solid. Due to the complex geometry of skull, brain and CSF, these were meshed with tetrahedral elements. The YEAHM is constituted by a total of 991617 second order ten-node tetrahedrons. More details about the mesh are presented in Table 2.1.

Table 2.1 YEAHM's mesh info

Part	Number of elements	Number of nodes
Skull	57257	14443
CSF	98032	27499
Brain	836328	153749

In order to verify the mesh influence, a mesh convergence analysis was carried out by varying the mesh density. Mesh convergence is used to check how small the element size should be to ensure that simulation results are unaffected by a further refinement. Basically, ensuring the best solution and consuming the minimal computational resources as possible. The mesh was considered converged when there was a negligible change in the numerical solution with further mesh refinement. In addition, some quality mesh measures were also assessed by tools available in ABAQUS, including the aspect ratio, shape factor, tri-face corner angles and edge size. Stable time increment was always used a criterion when verifying the elements.

Special attention was also given to volumetric locking. Tetrahedral elements may show volumetric locking, especially in case of soft tissues such as the brain, which are modelled as almost incompressible materials (Miller and Chinzei 2002). Thus, artificial stiffening due to incompressibility was always a concern. Therefore, a very refined mesh was used and a comparison was made between linear and quadratic tetrahedral elements. This comparison and the volumetric locking assessment are presented in the next chapter.

Modelling of YEAHM is a nonlinear problem, which involves finite deformations, nonlinear material models, complex loading and boundary conditions and geometric nonlinearity. In order to perform a feasible numerical simulation, a correct geometry must be used but that is not enough. Material properties should be previously assigned to the model and special attention must be taken regarding the boundary conditions and the interactions between the various structures of the model.

2.2.3 Material Modelling

Most biologic materials have nonlinear behaviour. In order to accurately simulate the brain response to loading conditions, accurate constitutive models must be used. Experimental data to identify the parameters for the constitutive models are also necessary.

The fidelity of FEHM models is highly dependent on the accuracy of the material properties used to model biological tissues (Rashid et al. 2012a). Depending on the application, viscoelastic and even purely elastic models have been used by various research groups. The most appropriate constitutive model that can be used to describe brain tissue will depend heavily on the topic of interest (Bilston 2011).

The characteristic time scale is very important when choosing a material model (Rashid et al. 2012a). In the case of head impact, the duration is usually of the order of milliseconds. Therefore, brain tissue must be characterised with properties over the expected range of loading rate appropriate for potentially injurious circumstances (Rashid et al. 2012a). Strain rates in the range of $10–100 \text{ s}^{-1}$ and compressive strain levels of 10–50% are the ones of direct relevance to impact injury (Bayly et al. 2006; Margulies et al. 1990; Meaney and Thibault 1990; Morrison et al. 2006). These are the ones used by Rashid et al. (2012a) to characterize brain tissue and used in this work to model the brain. Although the brain tissue samples tested by Rashid et al.

(2012a) were from porcine, Nicolle et al. (2005) and Thibault and Margulies (1998) observed no significant difference between the mechanical properties of human and porcine brain matter. Thus, the properties of porcine brain tissue may be used in the modelling of the human brain.

Rashid et al. (2012a, b) determined the mechanical properties of fresh brain tissue by performing unconfined compression tests and tensile tests at strains rates up to 90 s^{-1} and strains up to 30% and also relaxation tests to determine the time dependent material parameters. Although these tests were performed at 23 °C, the mechanical properties of brain tissue in unconfined compression are not affected significantly by variations in test temperatures (22–37 °C) (Rashid et al. 2012c).

Rashid et al. (2012a) found a significant increase in elastic moduli with the increase in strain rate, which confirms rate dependency. Cheng and Bilston (2007), Tamura et al. (2007) and Pervin and Chen (2009) covered a broad range of loading rates and also found that brain tissue was strain-rate sensitive.

Failure or tissue yield in shear appears to begin at approximately 100–200% strain at low-to-moderate loading rates (Bilston et al. 2001). This is a significantly higher strain than the one brain can withstand in tension and compression (Bilston 2011). Reports indicate failure for peak strains up to 30–50% and 20–60% for compression and tension, respectively (Bilston 2011). Thus, in this work, experimental data from compression and tensile tests were used to model the brain.

In summary, brain tissue is a very soft, strain rate sensitive, nonlinear viscoelastic material. It is usually assumed to be incompressible, or nearly incompressible, due to its very high water content (Brands et al. 2004; Miller and Chinzei 1997). Franceschini et al. (2006) subjected brain tissue to different conditions of hydration and verified brain's tissue incompressibility.

In this research, it is used a hyperelastic model to describe the nonlinear elasticity, combined with a viscoelastic model to describe the time-dependent behaviour. Both hyperelastic and viscoelastic material laws were already used to describe the brain's behaviour (Horgan and Gilchrist 2003; Miller et al. 2000; van Dommelen 2011). Thus, a hyper-viscoelastic material model is used to simulate brain tissue.

As for the hyperfoam model, the generic hyperelastic model is defined by a strain energy potential, also known as strain energy density function, which defines the strain energy stored in the material per unit of reference volume (initial volume) as function of the strain in the material. Each hyperelastic model has their own strain energy potential, W, from which the relationship between stress and strain tensors is derived. The strain energy function, W, is usually defined in terms of the invariants (I_1, I_2, I_3) of the strain tensor, which is itself defined by the deformation gradient tensor, $\boldsymbol{F}$. This relation is established by the left Cauchy-Green deformation tensor, $\boldsymbol{B}$:

$$\boldsymbol{B} = \boldsymbol{F}\boldsymbol{F}^T \tag{2.1}$$

The invariants of B are defined as:

$$I_1 = \text{tr}(B) = \lambda_1^2 + \lambda_2^2 + \lambda_3^2$$
$$I_2 = \frac{1}{2}[\text{tr}(B)^2 - \text{tr}(B^2)] = \lambda_1^2\lambda_2^2 + \lambda_2^2\lambda_3^2 + \lambda_1^2\lambda_3^2 \qquad (2.2)$$
$$I_3 = \det B = J^2 = (\det(F))^2 = \lambda_1^2\lambda_2^2\lambda_3^2$$

where λ_i are the principal stretches and J is the total volume ratio given by the determinant of the deformation gradient. The Ogden model (Ogden 1972) has been used in the past to describe the nonlinear mechanical behaviour of the brain, as well as of other nonlinear soft tissues (Brittany and Margulies 2006; Lin et al. 2008; Miller and Chinzei 2002; Prange and Margulies 2002; Velardi et al. 2006). Soft biological tissue is often modelled with success by the Ogden hyperelastic function:

$$W = \sum_{i=1}^{N} \frac{2\mu_i}{\alpha_i^2}(\bar{\lambda}_1^{\alpha_i} + \bar{\lambda}_2^{\alpha_i} + \bar{\lambda}_3^{\alpha_i} - 3) + \sum_{i=1}^{N} \frac{1}{D_i}(J - 1)^{2i} \qquad (2.3)$$

where $\bar{\lambda}_i$ are the deviatoric principal stretches, which can be obtained through the relation between the total volume ratio J and the the principal stretches λ_i,

$$\bar{\lambda}_i = J^{-1/3}\lambda_i \qquad (2.4)$$

N, μ_i, α_i and D_i are material parameters. The initial shear modulus can be obtained through:

$$\mu_0 = \sum_{i=1}^{N} \mu_i \qquad (2.5)$$

The bulk modulus for the Ogden form is given by:

$$K_0 = \frac{2}{D_1} \qquad (2.6)$$

Thus, the one-term Ogden hyperelastic function is given by:

$$W = \frac{2\mu_0}{\alpha_1^2}(\bar{\lambda}_1^{\alpha_1} + \bar{\lambda}_2^{\alpha_1} + \bar{\lambda}_3^{\alpha_1} - 3) + \frac{1}{D_1}(J - 1)^2 \qquad (2.7)$$

If a material is incompressible, the third strain invariant has a value of 1, and the strain energy function is only a function of the first two invariants. Thus, an isotropic hyperelastic incompressible material is characterised by a strain-energy density function W, which is a function of two principal strain invariants only. The stress-strain relationship is then obtained from a partial derivative of the strain energy potential with respect to deformation gradient tensor F.

Table 2.2 Properties used to model the brain

ρ [kg/m³]	μ [MPa]	α_1	D_1 [MPa⁻¹]	g_1	g_2	τ_1 [s]	τ_2 [s]
1040	0.012	5.0507	0.04	0.5837	0.2387	0.02571	0.02570

The elastic and viscoelastic behaviour of brain tissue can be characterised using an Ogden based nonlinear viscoelastic model (Rashid et al. 2012a). The relaxation response is based on a Prony series and the strain energy function is developed in the form of a convolution integral, already used by some research groups (Rashid et al. 2012a; Miller and Chinzei 2002; Prange and Margulies 2002).

Thus, in order to model the brain's nonlinear elasticity and the time-dependent behaviour, the one-term Ogden hyperelastic model and a Prony-series are combined:

$$W = \frac{2}{\alpha_1^2} \int_0^t [\mu(t-\tau)\frac{d}{d\tau}(\bar{\lambda}_1^{\alpha_1} + \bar{\lambda}_2^{\alpha_1} + \bar{\lambda}_3^{\alpha_1} - 3)]d\tau + \frac{1}{D_1}(J-1)^2 \quad (2.8)$$

Hence, the relaxation of the time-dependent shear modulus $\mu(t)$ to describe the viscous response of the tissue is:

$$\mu(t) = \mu_0[1 - \sum_{k=1}^n g_k(1 - e^{-t/\tau_k})] \quad (2.9)$$

where μ_0 is the initial shear modulus, τ_k are the characteristic relaxation times and g_k are the relaxation coefficients, which can be determined from the experimental data.

Rashid et al. (2012a, b) estimated optimal parameters for one-term Ogden model and for Prony series, which provided an excellent fitting to the experimental data. The parameters used in this research are based on the ones determined by Rashid et al. (2012a, b). Table 2.2 presents the values used to model the brain.

Mechanical properties of grey and white matter are expected to be different. Unfortunately, data reported in literature are not consistent in terms of which brain matter is stiffer than the other (Yang and King 2011). There is a lack of data about the mechanical properties on axonal directional dependency to justify the use of such a computationally expensive representation (Yang and King 2011). Limited by CPU power, it is also not practical to model individual cells and axons at this stage. As a result, most head models assume the brain to be homogeneous and isotropic (Miller et al. 2011), as in this work.

Simulations with CSF modelled as fluid were performed, but the required computational resources to simulate it were excessive. CSF was modelled as a solid with a very low shear modulus and as a hyperelastic material, using the Mooney-Rivlin strain energy potential:

$$W = C_{10}(\bar{I}_1 - 3) + C_{01}(\bar{I}_2 - 3) + \frac{1}{D_1}(J-1)^2 \quad (2.10)$$

where W is the strain energy per unit of reference volume; C_{10}, C_{01}, and D_1 are material parameters; and $\bar{I}_1$ and $\bar{I}_2$ are the first and second deviatoric strain invariants defined as:

$$\bar{I}_1 = J^{-2/3} I_1 \tag{2.11}$$

$$\bar{I}_2 = J^{-4/3} I_2 \tag{2.12}$$

The bulk modulus can be obtained through the Eq. 2.6. The initial shear modulus is given by:

$$\mu_0 = 2(C_{10} + C_{01}) \tag{2.13}$$

Table 2.3 gives the values used to model the CSF. The CSF density used is the same as water since the two are similar. Regarding the values used for the C_{10}, C_{01} and D_1, these are higher than the ones typically used in the literature. This is normal since YEAHM's CSF global model needs to account for all the internal contents, except the brain. Nevertheless, the relation $C_{10} = 0.9\, C_{01}$ used by Gilchrist (2003) was here adopted.

Skull bone is usually modelled as linear elastic and isotropic material, which is considered a reasonable approximation (Kleiven 2002). In this work, it was also modelled as an isotropic linear elastic material. Table 2.4 gives the values used to model the bone, where ρ, E and ν are the density, Young's modulus and Poisson's ratio, respectively.

Given the complexity and strong nonlinearity of brain tissue mechanical response, it is unrealistic to expect that one constitutive model will fit all circumstances. Depending on the loading regimes, specific brain tissue properties may be necessary to capture the correct response of brain tissue. Fortunately, the following tests performed in cadavers and used for validation were designed to replicate road accidents.

Table 2.3 Properties used to model the CSF

ρ [kg/m^3]	C_{10} [MPa]	C_{01} [MPa]	D_1 [MPa^{-1}]
1000	0.9	1	0.9

Table 2.4 Properties used to model the skull

ρ [kg/m^3]	E [MPa]	ν
1800	6000	0.21

2.2.4 Contact and Boundary Conditions

During a head impact, CSF makes it possible for brain to move relatively to the skull. A great number of researchers fix the brain surface to the skull, sharing the nodes or even creating a rigid connection. This is not biofidelic and the best alternative is to allow the motion between brain and skull.

In order to correctly simulate the brain response upon impact and mimic experimental test conditions, appropriate boundary conditions must be applied. The relative motion between the skull and brain is simulated by the sliding interface between the skull and CSF and between the CSF and brain. Finite sliding formulation and kinematic contact method were used with a friction coefficient for tangential behaviour of 0.2 as used in Horgan and Gilchrist (2004) and proposed by Miller et al. (1998). More details about the modelling of YEAHM can be found in Fernandes et al. (2018).

References

P.V. Bayly, E.E. Black, R. Pedersen et al., In vivo imaging of rapid deformation and strain in an animal model of traumatic brain injury. J. Biomech. **39**, 1086–1095 (2006)

L.E. Bilston, Z. Liu, N. Phan-Thien, Large strain behaviour of brain tissue in shear: some experimental data and differential constitutive model. Biorheology **38**, 335–345 (2001)

L.E. Bilston, Brain tissue mechanical properties, in *Biomechanics of the Brain*, ed. by K. Miller (Springer, New York, 2011), pp. 69–89

D.W.A. Brands, G.W.M. Peters, P.H.M. Bovendeerd, Design and numerical implementation of a 3-D non-linear viscoelastic constitutive model for brain tissue during impact. J. Biomech. **37**, 127–134 (2004)

C. Brittany, S.S. Margulies, Material properties of porcine parietal cortex. J. Biomech. **39**, 2521–2525 (2006)

CATIA V5, User's Manual. Dassault Systems (2008)

S. Cheng, L.E. Bilston, Unconfined compression of white matter. J. Biomech. **40**, 117–124 (2007)

P. Cignoni, M. Callieri, M. Corsini, M. Dellepiane, F. Ganovelli, G. Ranzuglia, MeshLab: an open-source mesh processing tool, in *Eurographics Italian Chapter Conference*, vol. 73 (2008), pp. 45–46

M. Claessens, F. Sauren, J. Wismans, Modeling of the human head under impact conditions: a parametric study. SAE Transactions Paper No. 973338 (1997), pp. 3829–3848

R.J.H. Cloots, H.M.T. Gervaise, J.A.W. van Dommelen, M.G.D. Geers, Biomechanics of traumatic brain injury: influences of the morphologic heterogeneities of the cerebral cortex. Ann. Biomed. Eng. **36**(7), 1203–1215 (2008)

R.J.H. Cloots, J.A.W. van Dommelen, S. Kleiven, M.G.D. Geers, Traumatic brain injury at multiple length scales: relating diffuse axonal injury to discrete axonal impairment, in *Proceedings of IRCOBI Conference*, Hanover, Germany (2010), pp. 119–130

F.A.O. Fernandes, R.J. Alves de Sousa, Head injury predictors in sports trauma—A state-of-the-art review. J. Eng. Med. **229**(8), 592–608 (2015)

F.A.O. Fernandes, D. Tchepel, R.J. Alves de Sousa, M. Ptak, Development and validation of a new finite element human head model-YEt Another Head Model (YEAHM). Engineering Computations **35**(1), 477–496 (2018)

G. Franceschini, D. Bigoni, P. Regitnig, G.A. Holzapfel, Brain tissue deforms similarly to filled elastomers and follows consolidation theory. J. Mech. Phys. Solids **54**(12), 2592–2620 (2006)

M.D. Gilchrist, Modelling and accident reconstruction of head impact injuries. Key Eng. Mater. **245–246**, 417–432 (2003)

M.D. Gilchrist, D. O'Donoghue, Simulation of the development of frontal head impact injury. Comput. Mech. **26**, 229–235 (2000)

E.S. Gurdjian, H.R. Lissner, V.R. Hodgson et al., Mechanisms of head injury. Clin. Neurosurg. **12**, 112–128 (1966)

W.N. Hardy, C.D. Foster, M.J. Mason, K.H. King, A.I. King, S. Tashman, Investigation of head injury mechanisms using neutral density technology and high-speed biplanar X-ray. Stapp Car Crash J. **45**, 337–368 (2001)

J. Ho, S. Kleiven, Dynamic response of the brain with vasculature: a three-dimensional computational study. J. Biomech. **40**, 3006–3012 (2007)

J. Ho, S. Kleiven, Can sulci protect the brain from traumatic injury? J. Biomech. **42**, 2074–2080 (2009)

T.J. Horgan, M.D. Gilchrist, The creation of three-dimensional finite element models for simulating head impact biomechanics. Int. J. Crashworthiness **8**(4), 353–366 (2003)

T.J. Horgan, M.D. Gilchrist, Influence of FE model variability in predicting brain motion and intracranial pressure changes in head impact simulations. Int. J. Crashworthiness **9**(4), 401–418 (2004)

J. Ivarsson, D.C. Viano, P. Lövsund, Influence of the lateral ventricles and irregular skull base on brain kinematics due to sagittal plane head rotation. J. Biomech. Eng. **124**, 422–431 (2002)

S. Kleiven, Finite element modeling of the human head. Doctoral Thesis, Technical Report, School of Technology an Health, Royal Institute of Technology, Stockholm, Sweden, 2002

S. Kleiven, Influence of direction and duration of impacts to the human head evaluated using the finite element method, in *Proceedings of IRCOBI Conference*, Prague, Czech Republic (2005), pp. 41–57

S. Kleiven, Predictors for traumatic brain injuries evaluated through accident reconstructions, in *Proceedings of the 51st Stapp Car Crash Conference* (2007), pp. 81–114

C. Lauret, M. Hrapko, J.A.W. van Dommelen, G.W.M. Peters, J.S.H.M. Wismans, Optical characterization of acceleration-induced strain fields in inhomogeneous brain slices. Med. Eng. Phys. **31**, 392–399 (2009)

D.C. Lin, D.I. Shreiber, E.K. Dimitriadis, F. Horkay, Spherical indentation of soft matter beyond the Hertzian regime: numerical and experimental validation of hyperelastic models. Biomech. Model. Mechanobiol. **8**, 345–358 (2008)

H. Mao, L. Zhang, B. Jiang et al., Development of a finite element human head model partially validated with thirty five experimental cases. J. Biomechan. Eng. **135**, 111002–15 (2013)

S.S. Margulies, L.E. Thibault, T.A. Gennarelli, Physical model simulations of brain injury in the primate. J. Biomech. **23**(8), 823–836 (1990)

D.F. Meaney, L.E. Thibault, Physical model studies of cortical brain deformation in response to high strain rate inertial loading, in *International Conference on the Biomechanics of Impacts. IRCOBI*, Lyon, France (1990)

Meshmixer manual. Autodesk (2012)

K. Miller, *Biomechanics of the Brain* (Springer, New York, 2011)

K. Miller, K. Chinzei, Constitutive modelling of brain tissue: experiment and theory. J. Biomech. **30**, 1115–1121 (1977)

K. Miller, K. Chinzei, Mechanical properties of brain tissue in tension. J. Biomech. **35**, 483–490 (2002)

R.T. Miller, S.S. Margulies, M. Leoni, M. Nonaka, X.H. Chen, D.H. Smith, D.F. Meaney, Finite element modeling approaches for predicting injury in an experimental model of severe diffuse axonal injury, in *Proceedings of 42nd Stapp Car Crash Conference*, SAE Paper 983154 (1998), pp. 155–166

K. Miller, K. Chinzei, G. Orssengo et al., Mechanical properties of brain tissue in-vivo: experiment and computer simulation. J. Biomech. **33**, 1369–1376 (2000)

K. Miller, A. Wittek, G. Joldes, Biomechanical modeling of the brain for computer-assisted neuro-surgery, in *Biomechanics of the Brain*, ed. by K. Miller (Springer, New York, 2011), pp. 111–136

B.I. Morrison, H.L. Cater, C.D. Benham, L.E. Sundstrom, An in vitro model of traumatic brain injury utilizing two-dimensional stretch of organotypic hippocampal slice cultures. J. Neurosci. Methods **150**, 192–201 (2006)

A.M. Nahum, R. Smith, C.C. Ward, Intracranial pressure dynamics during head impact, in *Proceeding of 21st Stapp Car Crash Conference* (1977), pp. 339–366

S. Nicolle, M. Lounis, R. Willinger, J.F. Palierne, Shear linear behaviour of brain tissue over a large frequency range. Biorheology **42**, 209–223 (2005)

R.W. Ogden, Large deformation isotropic elasticity-on the correlation of theory and experiment for incompressible rubber like solids. Proc. R. Soc. Lond. A. Math. Phys. Sci. **326**, 565–584 (1972)

A.K. Ommaya, R.L. Grubb, R.A. Naumann, Coup and contrecoup injury: observations on the mechanics of visible brain injuries in the rhesus monkey. J. Neurosurg. **35**, 503–516 (1971)

Osirix user manual. Pixmeo (2003)

F. Pervin, W.W. Chen, Dynamic mechanical response of bovine gray matter and white matter brain tissues under compression. J. Biomech. **42**, 731–735 (2009)

M.T. Prange, S.S. Margulies, Regional, directional, and age-dependent properties of the brain undergoing large deformation. J. Biomech. Eng. **124**(2), 244–252 (2002)

B. Rashid, M. Destrade, M.D. Gilchrist, Mechanical characterization of brain tissue in compression at dynamic strain rates. J. Mech. Behav. Biomed. Mater. **10**, 23–38 (2012a)

B. Rashid, M. Destrade, M.D. Gilchrist, Hyperelastic and viscoelastic properties of brain tissue in tension, in *Proceedings of the ASME 2012 International Mechanical Engineering Congress & Exposition, IMECE2012*, Houston, Texas, USA (2012b), pp. 9–15

B. Rashid, M. Destrade, M.D. Gilchrist, Temperature effects on brain tissue in compression. J. Mech. Behav. Biomed. Mater. **14**, 113–118 (2012c)

J.S. Ruan, P. Prasad, Coupling of a finite element human head model with lumped parameter hybrid III dummy model: preliminary results. J. Neurotrauma **12**(4), 725–734 (1995)

J. Ruan, P. Prasad, The effects of skull thickness variations on human head dynamic impact responses. Stapp Car Crash J. **45**, 395–414 (2001)

D. Sahoo, C. Deck, R. Willinger, Development and validation of an advanced anisotropic visco-hyperelastic human brain FE model. J. Mech. Behav. Biomed. Mater. **33**, 24–42 (2014)

E.G. Takhounts, S.A. Ridella, V. Hasija, R.E. Tannous, J.Q. Campbell, D. Malone, K. Danelson, J. Stitzel, S. Rowson, S. Duma, Investigation of traumatic brain injuries using the next generation of simulated injury monitor (SIMon) finite element head model. Stapp Car Crash J. **52**, 1–31 (2008)

A. Tamura, S. Hayashi, I. Watanabe et al., Mechanical characterization of brain tissue in high-rate compression. J. Biomech. Sci. Eng. **2**, 115–126 (2007)

K.L. Thibault, S.S. Margulies, Age-dependent material properties of the porcine cerebrum: effect on pediatric inertial head injury criteria. J. Biomech. **31**, 1119–1126 (1998)

K. Tse, S. Lim, V. Tan, H. Lee, A review of head injury and finite element head models. Am. J. Eng. Technol. Soc. **1**(5), 28–52 (2014)

J. van Dommelen, Constitutive modelling of brain tissue for prediction of traumatic brain injury. Neural Tissue Biomech. **3**, 41–67 (2011)

F. Velardi, F. Fraternali, M. Angelillo, Anisotropic constitutive equations and experimental tensile behavior of brain tissue. Biomech. Model. Mechanobiol. **5**, 53–61 (2006)

J. Yang Investigation of brain trauma biomechanics in vehicle traffic accidents using human body computational models. in *Computational Biomechanics for Medicine: Soft Tissues and the Musculoskeletal System*, ed. by A. Wittek et al. (Springer Science+Business Media LLC, 2011)

K.H. Yang, A.I. King, Modeling of the brain for injury simulation and prevention, in *Biomechanics of the Brain*, ed. by K. Miller (Springer, New York, 2011), pp. 91–110

L. Zhang, K. Yang, R. Dwarampudi, K. Omori, T. Li, K. Chang, W.N. Hardy, T.B. Khalil, A.I. King, Recent advances in brain injury research: a new human head model development and validation. Stapp Car Crash J. **45**, 369–394 (2001)

L. Zhang, J. Bae, W.N. Hardy et al., Computational study of the contribution of the vasculature on the dynamic response of the brain. Stapp Car Crash J. **46**, 145–164 (2002)

J. Zhang, N. Yoganandan, F.A. Pintar, Y. Guan, B. Shender, G. Paskoff, P. Laud, Effects of tissue preservation temperature on high strain-rate material properties of brain. J. Biomech. **44**, 391–396 (2011)

Chapter 3
Validation of YEAHM

3.1 Simulation of Impacts on Cadavers

Over the decades, a few studies were made on human cadavers. Some of these, which are considered benchmark tests, were used in this study to validate YEAHM. Experiments from Nahum et al. (1977) and Hardy et al. (2001) were used to assess YEAHM's intracranial pressure response and brain motion, respectively.

3.1.1 Intracranial Pressure Response Validation

Nahum et al. (1977) performed impacts by submitting rigid masses travelling at a constant velocity against stationary seated unembalmed cadavers. These type of tests and data are rare due to the nature of it. Nevertheless, these tests performed by Nahum et al. (1977) are today's reference for FEHM validation.

Careful storage of this type of experimental material together with testing soon after death were necessary in order to gather useful information (Fallenstein et al. 1969; Nahum and Smith 1976). Since the impacts were performed on cadavers, the authors of these experiments performed static fluid pressurization of the cranial vascular network and cerebral spinal fluid space to in vivo pressure levels at impact. According to Nahum and Smith (1976), the inability to study pathophysiologic changes and therefore, questions concerning the mechanisms of concussion are some of the disadvantages of using post mortem material. Nevertheless, the unembalmed cadaver could supply information regarding tissue changes that would be considered either lethal or reversible over an extended period of time in vivo and might be correlated with intra-operative or post mortem observations. In addition, in Nahum and Smith (1976), all of the tissue changes produced in the experimental specimens were observed in post mortem examination of in vivo head injury cases (Lindenberg and Freytag 1960).

In these tests, the head was not supported and it was not constrained. Thus, the head motion during impact was not influenced. The blow was delivered to the frontal bone in the mid-sagittal plane in an anterior-posterior direction. The skull was rotated

© The Author(s) 2018
F. A. O. Fernandes et al., *Head Injury Simulation in Road Traffic Accidents*, SpringerBriefs in Applied Sciences and Technology,
https://doi.org/10.1007/978-3-319-89926-8_3

Table 3.1 Cranial anthropometry comparison between experiment 37 and YEAHM

Subject	Age	A[mm]	B[mm]	C[mm]	D[mm]	E[mm]	F[mm]	G[mm]	H[mm]
Exp. 37	42	145	167	192	136	223	560	372	355
YEAHM	65	145	169	186	133	223	559	349	351

A—Head breadth (maximum above ears)   E—Head height (gnathion to vertex)
B—Head length (inion to glabella)   F—Head circumference (max. forehead, over ears)
C—Head length (ophistocranon to glabella)   G—Head midsagittal arc length (inion to glabella)
D—Head height (tragus to top of head)   H—Head coronal arc length (tragus to tragus)

forward so that the Frankfort anatomical plane was inclined 45° to the horizontal. Various padding materials were interposed between the skull and impactor to obtain the proper impact duration.

The experiment selected to validate YEAHM, experiment 37, is the most used in the literature to validate FEHMs. In addition, the subject of this experiment has the closest cranial anthropometric measurements to YEAHM. These measurements are described in Table 3.1. Both, the experiment 37 and the volunteer from who the medical images were obtained, are male subjects. A lateral view of an adult human skull, indicating the Frankfort anatomical plane and the cranial landmarks used in the anthropometric measurements, is shown in Fig. 3.1.

In experiment 37, a cylindrical mass of 5.59 kg hit the subject at 9.94 m/s. Figure 3.1 illustrates the configuration for simulation of the head impact test. The boundary conditions of simulation were defined based on test configurations. The impactor was defined as rigid, and the padding material in its front end was modelled as a linear elastic material with a Young's modulus of 6 MPa and a Poisson's ratio of 0.16.

The impact duration is so short that the neck has no effect on head response in this time window. Nahum et al. (1977) observed that dynamic pressure changes within the skull had ceased before significant rotation of the skull had occurred. Thus, a free boundary condition was assumed. ABAQUS Explicit solver with the large deformation option was used to simulate the impacts.

The validation consists in the simulation of experiment 37 performed by Nahum et al. (1977), which is the reference for FEHMs validation. In these experiments, the input force and the intracranial pressure-time histories were recorded. Transducers were placed in the frontal bone adjacent to the impact contact area, immediately posterior and superior to the coronal and squamosal sutures respectively in the parietal bone, and inferior to the lambdoidal suture in the occipital bone. Additionally, transducers were placed in the occipital bone at the posterior fossa. In the selected experiment, bilateral occipital pressures were also monitored. Thus, the contact force between the impactor and the head, and the pressure in five different positions were used in YEAHM's validation. An illustration of the regions used by Nahum et al. (1977) to measure the pressure is shown in Fig. 3.2.

In order to validate YEAHM, the results from simulation and from experiment 37 are compared in Figs. 3.3, 3.4, 3.5, 3.6, 3.7 and 3.8. These show the contact

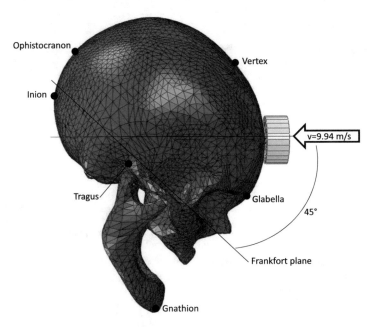

Fig. 3.1 Configuration of Nahum experiment for model validation. Anatomic landmarks used in craniometric measurements '

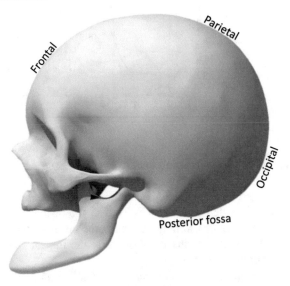

Fig. 3.2 Regions where pressure was measured by Nahum et al. (1977)

force between the impactor and the head, frontal pressure, parietal pressure, occipital pressures and posterior fossa pressure, respectively.

Fig. 3.3 Comparison of input force between experimental and simulation results

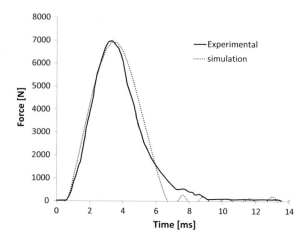

Fig. 3.4 Comparison of frontal pressure between experimental and simulation results

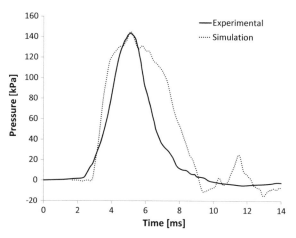

Nahum et al. (1977) recorded high positive peak pressures beneath the impact site in the frontal region. The same was observed in the simulations with YEAHM. The pressure decreased and eventually became negative as the area opposite to the blow was approached, which was also observed in the results of the simulations. The greatest negative pressures were generated at the posterior fossa, which due to the inclination of the skull, was the point opposite the impact site. This was also observed in the simulations with YEAHM.

There is a reasonable agreement between the results computed with YEAHM and the ones reported by Nahum et al. (1977). In this simulation of a blunt impact to a stationary head, it was clear the faster movement from skull relatively to the brain, which originated a pressure gradient. Upon the impact, the skull and the brain tend to relatively move towards the impact site creating an area of elevated pressure where the intracranial tissues are compressed. This is known as coup and opposite

Fig. 3.5 Comparison of parietal pressure between experimental and simulation results

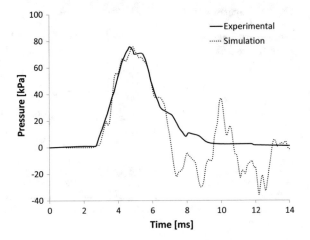

Fig. 3.6 Comparison of occipital pressure between experimental and simulation results

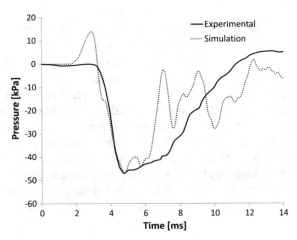

Fig. 3.7 Comparison of occipital pressure between experimental and simulation results

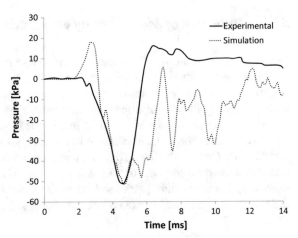

Fig. 3.8 Comparison of
posterior fossa pressure
between experimental and
simulation results

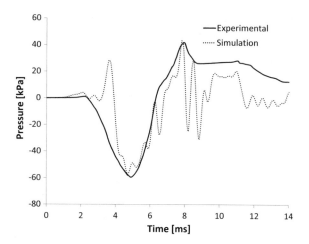

to it, where brain tissues are stretched and under negative pressures, is known as
contrecoup contusion (Chinn and Hynd 2009). Figures 3.9 and 3.10 illustrate pressure
gradients across the brain, showing the coup and contrecoup phenomenons during
the simulation of Nahum's experiment.

Some discrepancies observed in the previous figures may be explained by several
factors. According to Bilston (2011), tests with fresh and post-mortem tissues may
give different results. Also, some internal contents, such as the meninges, were not
modelled separately, which may have influenced the results. Nevertheless, the results
from the simulations were good enough to consider YEAHM validated. Actually,
comparing these results with the ones from state-of-the-art models available in the
literature, the YEAHM results are quite good. Thus, the intracranial pressure of
YEAHM is considered validated.

3.1.2 Influence of Mesh Quality on the Results

Due to complex geometry of the human head, the semi-automatic hexahedral mesh
generation was a challenging problem. Therefore, the tetrahedral mesh was used.
Regrettably, the standard formulation of the linear tetrahedral element exhibits volumetric locking in case of almost incompressible materials (Joldes et al. 2009).
The standard linear tetrahedral element in Abaqus (constant stress, 3D, 4-node i.e.
C3D4) calculates the element pressure in the expression of the volumetric internal
virtual work. On the other hand, this element is not prone to hourglassing. Thus, special attention was also given to volumetric locking as inauthentic pressure stresses
develop at the integration point level, causing an element to behave too stiffly for
deformations that should cause no volume changes. In this case, the finite element

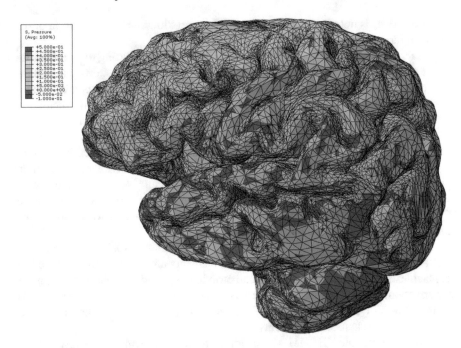

Fig. 3.9 Coup phenomenon (hydrostatic pressure [MPa])

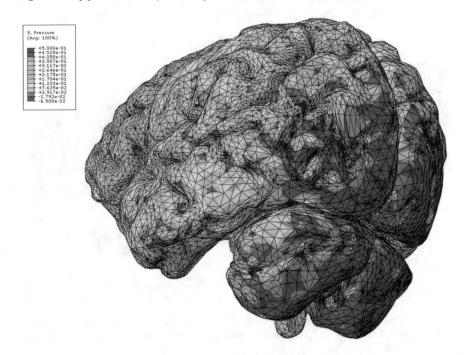

Fig. 3.10 Contrecoup phenomenon (hydrostatic pressure [MPa])

method (FEM) is not able to give a reasonable approximation to the solution of the problem (de Souza Neto et al. 1996).

In fact, the volumetric locking phenomenon was detected during the simulations when C3D4 element was used to model the CSF and brain, as shown previously. The pressure values—quilt-style contour plot—presented a "checkerboard" pattern depicted in Fig. 3.11. The pressure values changed considerably from one integration point to the other—clearing proving that volumetric locking was occurring.

Some different solutions have been proposed over the time to prevent the locking. Some of which constant dilatation, assumed strain are specialized in preventing dilatation locking and others reduced integration, selective reduced integration, Herrmann formulation, average nodal pressure (ANP) can also prevent other types of locking as volume locking (Miller et al. 2011). In this particular case, it was used C3D10M elements (constant stress, 3D, 10-node modified element) to replace the linear tetrahedral elements, standard C3D4.

The C3D10M elements use a lumped matrix formulation for dynamic analysis (ABAQUS 2010). The modified tetrahedral elements are reported to work well in contact, exhibit minimal shear and volumetric locking, and are robust during finite deformation. When the hourglass control is chosen, the hourglass modes in C3D10M elements do not usually propagate. Thus, the hourglass stiffness is usually not as significant as for first-order elements.

In order to validate YEAHM with quadratic tetrahedral elements, the results from simulation and from Nahum's experiment 37 are compared in Figs. 3.12, 3.13, 3.14, 3.15, 3.16, 3.17. These show the contact force between head and impactor, frontal

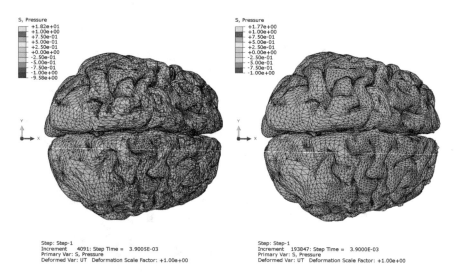

Fig. 3.11 Checkerboard pattern on the brain model while using C3D4 elements (left) versus improved model meshed with C3D10M elements (right)—quilt-style contour plot of hydrostatic pressure [MPa]

pressure, parietal pressure, occipital pressures and posterior fossa pressure, respectively.

Again, there is reasonable agreement between the results from the simulation and the ones reported by Nahum et al. (1977). In terms of brain pressure gradient the results were also similar. Figures 3.18 and 3.19 illustrate pressure gradients across the brain, showing the coup and contrecoup phenomenons during the simulation of Nahum's experiment with quadratic tetrahedral elements.

This finite element mesh comparison shows the importance of a careful choice of finite element formulations to model some of the head parts constituted by materials with an incompressible behaviour. Indeed, locking phenomena may appear for low order elements and spoil a whole head model.

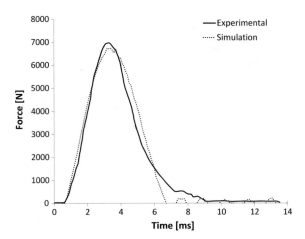

Fig. 3.12 Comparison of input force between experimental and numerical results

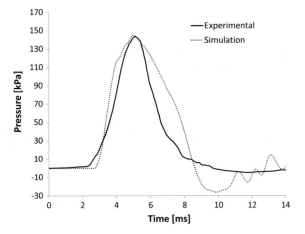

Fig. 3.13 Comparison of frontal pressure between experimental and numerical results

Fig. 3.14 Comparison of parietal pressure between experimental and numerical results

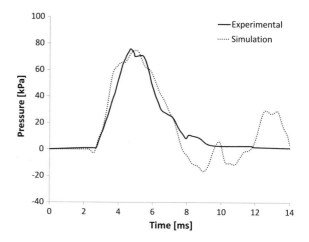

Fig. 3.15 Comparison of occipital pressure between experimental and numerical results

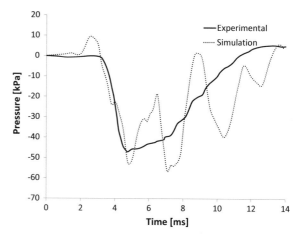

Fig. 3.16 Comparison of occipital pressure between experimental and numerical results

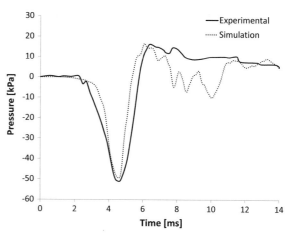

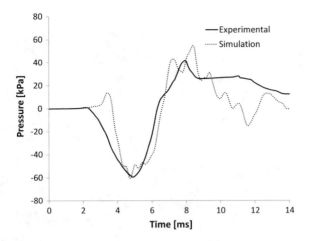

Fig. 3.17 Comparison of fossa pressure between experimental and numerical results

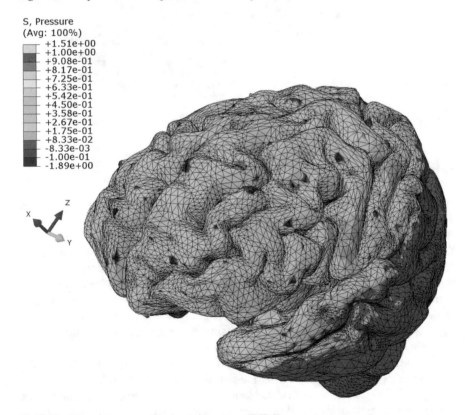

Fig. 3.18 Coup phenomenon (hydrostatic pressure [MPa])

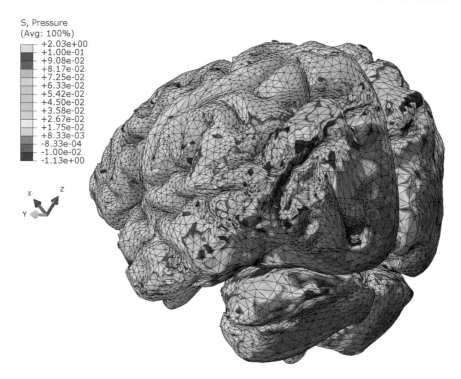

Fig. 3.19 Contrecoup phenomenon (hydrostatic pressure [MPa]—reversed colour spectrum)

3.1.3   Brain Motion Validation

In addition to the experiments performed by Nahum et al. (1977), experiments from Hardy et al. (2001) are also used by other authors to validate their models. This is usually done to validate the motion of the brain model. One of these experiments is the C755-T2. It is an occipital impact with a velocity of 2 m/s. In these experiments, the local brain motion was measured by tracking neutral-density targets (NDTs), using a high-speed biplanar X-ray system during different impact conditions. The NDTs were implanted in two vertical columns, a posterior and an anterior columns located at the occipito-parietal and the temporo-parietal regions respectively, as shown in Fig. 3.20. In the coronal plane, the two columns were approximately aligned with the right eye.

The head model nodes nearest located to the position of the NDTs were used to validate the brain response during numerical replication of the test. In addition, Hardy et al. (2001) measured the head kinematics (all six degrees of freedom, three components of translational and rotational acceleration) during impact. The exactly same kinematics measured by Hardy et al. (2001) during the C755-T2 experiment, were applied to the local coordinate system attached to the YEAHM's COG, which

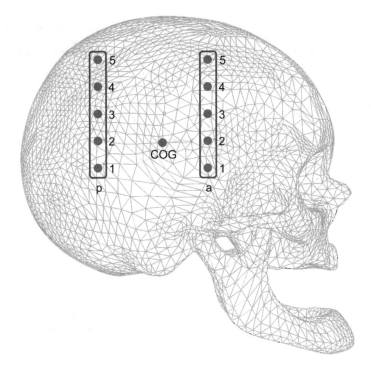

Fig. 3.20 Illustration of the NDTs columns location used to track brain motion

is the origin and a reference point of the skull. The latter was modelled as rigid for this validation and the local coordinate system moves with it. Modelling the skull as a rigid part in this specific case, it is considered a feasible simplification due to the absence of skull fracture and considerable deformations. In addition, the skull bone is much stiffer than brain matter and thus, modelling it with a much higher Young's modulus or as a rigid part is reasonably the same. Additionally, it is not simulated a direct impact. Instead, the translational and rotational accelerations measured by Hardy et al. (2001), were used as input for simulation of C755-T2 experiment. The data used to drive YEAHM are shown in Figs. 3.21 and 3.22.

The simulation for experiment C755-T2 was conducted and the brain motion data of the selected nodes were compared with experimental NDTs displacement. The simulation was conducted up to a duration of 60 ms, which is the duration of the experiments performed by Hardy et al. (2001).

YEAHM has been validated against the pressure data provided by Nahum et al. (1977). In order to further validate this model, validations were performed regarding brain motion from the experimental impacts performed in Hardy et al. (2001). The experiment C755-T2 from Hardy et al. (2001) was replicated with YEAHM.

The brain model nearest nodes to the position of NDTs were chosen to analyse the brain motion during the simulation. The simulation for experiment C755-T2

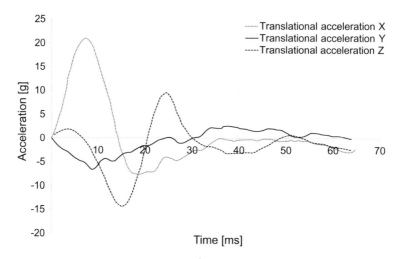

Fig. 3.21 Translational acceleration used as input for simulation of C755-T2 experiment

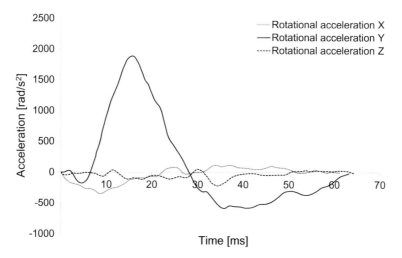

Fig. 3.22 Rotational acceleration used as input for simulation of C755-T2 experiment

was conducted and the brain motion data of selected nodes were compared with experimental NDTs relative displacement.

The simulation results for the relative displacement of five NDTs locations in X and Z directions for the occipital impact test C755-T2 and its comparison with experimental data are illustrated in Figs. 3.23 and 3.24. Figure 3.23 shows the displacement-time history for NDTs at the temporo-parietal region. Figure 3.24 shows the NDTs motion at the occipito-parietal location. In both figures, the left and right plots represent the NDTs relative displacement in the X and Z directions, respectively. The

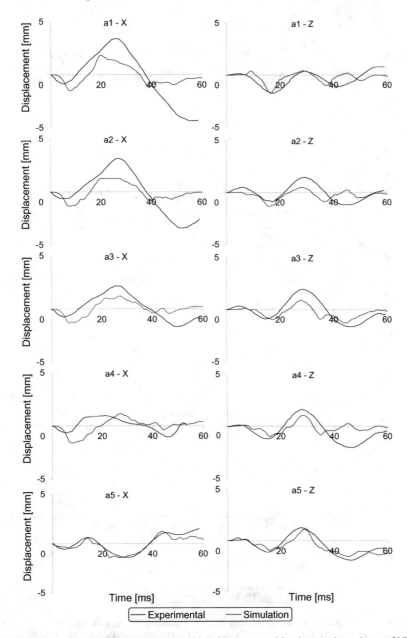

Fig. 3.23 Comparison of displacement-time histories, measured by the anterior column of NDTs located at the temporo-parietal region, between C755-T2 experiment and its simulation with YEAHM

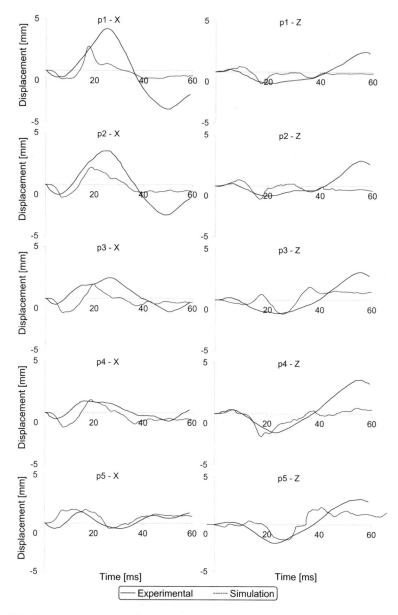

Fig. 3.24 Comparison of displacement-time histories, measured by the posterior column of NDTs located at the occipito-parietal region, between C755-T2 experiment and its simulation with YEAHM

motion pattern of the NDTs is typically characterised by maximum and minimum displacements which lay between 20 and 40 ms.

Although there are some differences between the experiments and the results from the simulations, Figs. 3.23 and 3.24 show that simulations are in accordance with the experimental data from the NDTs. In general, the simulated relative displacements are close to the experiments or at least follow the same trend. The major discrepancies found in these simulations with YEAHM were the maximum displacements in X direction for NDTs 1 and 2 in both anterior and posterior columns. In other words, the worst results computed with YEAHM were the relative displacements in X direction for NDTs a1, a2, p1 and p2. The source of this discrepancy could be the absence of a singular model for falx cerebri and cerebelli and tentorium cerebelli, instead of modelling everything as a CSF global model.

Nevertheless, these results were considered good enough to trust on YEAHM's brain motion response. In addition, by comparing the results of YEAHM with other FEHMs available in the literature and cited as state-of-the-art models in Chap. 1, excellent results were computed with YEAHM. Probably because the majority of these FEHMs have simplified brain geometries and a fixed brain surface to the skull.

In conclusion, in this chapter, a new FEHM was developed and validated against the cadaver impacts performed by Nahum et al. (1977) and Hardy et al. (2001). This model has a geometric accurate brain model, where sulci and gyri are present. In addition, relative motion between brain and skull is also possible with this model. YEAHM, associated with suitable head injury criteria, can be used in many applications, for instance in accidents reconstruction and in the design of helmets.

References

ABAQUS 6.10 documentation (Hibbitt, Karlsson & Sorensen, Inc., 2010)

L.E. Bilston, Brain tissue mechanical properties, in *Biomechanics of the Brain*, ed. by K. Miller (Springer, New York, 2011), pp. 69–89

B. Chinn, D. Hynd, *Technical Response to the Unpublished Paper: Critical Evaluation of the Sharp Motorcycle Helmet Rating* (TRL Published Project Report, 2009)

E.A. de Souza Neto, D. Peric, M. Dutko, D.R.J. Owen, Design of simple low order finite elements for large strain analysis of nearly incompressible solids. Int. J. Solids Struct. **33**(20), 3277–3296 (1996)

G. Fallenstein, V. Hulce, J. Melvin, Dynamic mechanical properties of human brain tissue. J. Biomech. **2**(3), 217–226 (1969)

W.N. Hardy, C.D. Foster, M.J. Mason, K.H. King, A.I. King, S. Tashman, Investigation of head injury mechanisms using neutral density technology and high-speed biplanar X-ray. Stapp Car Crash J. **45**, 337–368 (2001)

G.R. Joldes, A. Wittek, K. Miller, Non-locking tetrahedral finite element for surgical simulation. Commun. Numer. Methods Eng. **25**, 827–836 (2009)

R. Lindenberg, E. Freytag, The mechanism of cerebral contusions. A.M.A. Arch. Pathol. **69**, 440–469 (1960)

K. Miller, A. Wittek, G. Joldes, Biomechanical modeling of the brain for computer-assisted neurosurgery, in *Biomechanics of the Brain*, ed. by K. Miller (Springer, New York, 2011), pp. 111–136

A.M. Nahum, R. Smith, An experimental model for closed head impact injury. SAE Technical Paper 760825 (1976), pp. 2638–2651

A.M. Nahum, R. Smith, C.C. Ward, Intracranial pressure dynamics during head impact, in *Proceeding of 21st Stapp Car Crash Conference* (1977), pp. 339–366

Chapter 4
Application of Numerical Methods for Accident Reconstruction and Forensic Analysis

4.1 Introduction

Pedestrians and cyclists form the second largest group of road fatalities, around one-third of the seriously injured or killed vulnerable road users (VRU) in European Union (EU) (Simms et al. 2015; Ptak et al. 2012; European Commission 2015). Motorcyclist's share of all road deaths adds, on average in EU, 15% to this statistics (European Commission 2015). The disproportion in pedestrian/cyclist injuries and fatalities strongly correlates with roads and pavements infrastructure, speed limits and the national health care systems (Podvezko and Sivilevičius 2013; Nordfjærn and Zavareh 2016; Kadali and Vedagiri 2016; Asaithambi et al. 2016). Additionally, the examination of the mobility trends in the EU countries shows growth of walking and bicycle usage as a mean of transport. Many cities have seen a steady increase of their levels of cycling. In Paris, bicycle use has tripled in the last 10 years (Küster 2015). The fact that more people choose to walk or use a bike is essentially a good development for the EU and in line with the need for greener transport. Whereas cycling, e-cycling (electrical bicycle), bike-sharing schemes and walking start playing a major role in personal mobility in EU, the safety countermeasures are not sufficient (Supreame Audit Office 2016).

In Fig. 4.1, the authors collated the data reported for 25 EU members, with an additional EU average, for pedestrians' and cyclists' share of all who died on EU roads. The percentage of cyclists killed correlates strongly with countries' bicycle tradition and proper infrastructure, which encourage inhabitants to choose a bicycle as a mean of transport. Thus, the higher than average shares are reported from the Netherlands and Denmark. On the other hand, the high share of pedestrian fatalities distinguishes relatively new EU Member States as in Romania, Latvia, Poland and Lithuania pedestrians contribute to more than 30% of all road deaths (European Commission 2015). However, an interesting correlation forms as we compare the road safety level in various countries (fatality rate per million inhabitants) with the pedestrian deaths on roads. For the majority of countries, the lower the overall fatality

© The Author(s) 2018
F. A. O. Fernandes et al., *Head Injury Simulation in Road Traffic Accidents*, SpringerBriefs in Applied Sciences and Technology, https://doi.org/10.1007/978-3-319-89926-8_4

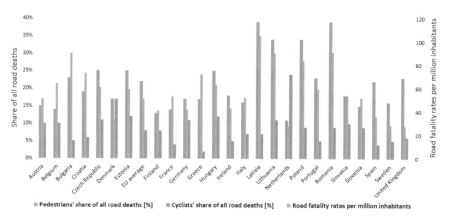

Fig. 4.1 Pedestrians' and cyclists' share of all road deaths [%] in contrast to road fatality rates per million inhabitants [-] in European Union in 2014 (based on data from European Commission (2015))

rate, the lower the pedestrians' fatality contribution. In other words, the percentage of pedestrians who are killed on the country's road may give an approximate idea about the general country's road safety.

Due to technological advances, it sounds feasible to implement systems aimed at accidents prevention or mitigation of impact speed by (semi)autonomous braking or avoidance manoeuvres—formally named as active safety systems. The leap forward in technology was possible when the informal, often mechanical connections between subsystems were replaced by systematic networking, steadily applied through the vehicle.

4.2 Vulnerable Road User Impact—Pedestrian Kinematics

Regarding car-to-pedestrian frontal impacts, 80% of the accidents may be classified into one of the five typical scenarios. The remaining 20% includes the pedestrian dragging circumstance, which is also depicted in Fig. 4.2 where the authors numerically simulated the phases of accidents basing on Simms et al. (2015) and Ptak et al. (2012). The mechanism of the impact was determined for the 50-percentile MAthematical DYnamic MOdeling (MADYMO) male dummy in the standing stance and struck from the side by a front of vehicle—this is a typical situation encompassing 80% car-to-pedestrian collisions (European Commission 2015; Podvezko and Sivilevičius 2013).

- Forward projection—takes place when an unprotected road user is struck by a flat surface of the vehicle front-end—typically heavy goods vehicles, buses, trucks. The vehicle hits the pedestrian above the centre of the body mass. The injuries of legs, hip and upper limbs occur almost simultaneously. During a collision, the vehicle and pedestrian speed equalise, causing sudden linear acceleration of the pedestrian body. The pedestrian does not gain significant angular velocity so the body is not to fold around the front-end. The elastic strain of the vehicle can result in pedestrian higher longitudinal speed relating to the vehicle, which often results in projection of the body from the vehicle. If the car is not sufficiently decelerated, the scenario is followed by secondary pedestrian overrun.

- Wrap projection—occurs when in the first phase pedestrian comes into contact with the front part of the vehicle, below pedestrian centre of mass. Lower limbs gain angular momentum that causes rotation in the direction of the bonnet. Because of the inertia of the individual body, which is not initially in contact with the vehicle, i.e. the head and torso, it remains immovable by at least 30 ms after the collision (Joldes et al. 2009). Subsequently, there is a contact between the bonnet leading edge and the upper part of the leg. During the next phase, the body wraps over the bonnet, followed by the chest and head struck against the hood, A-pillar or windshield—the rate of rotation depends on the degree of eccentricity of the contact and the impact speed. After the collision, the pedestrian body remains on the bonnet until the driver does not take intensively braking. Then, the limp body falls down on the road. If the vehicle is not braking adequately, the pedestrian can pass over the roof of the vehicle and land behind it—this is known as further described roof vault.
- Somersault—the situation starts similarly to the above warp projection. However, in this case, the pedestrian's legs are not at the front of the vehicle, the pedestrian shall be raised up, which is caused by a sufficiently large impact velocity and shape of the vehicle. Withholding legs rotate transitive to the car roof while the head remains on the bonnet. Further phases of the case are directly related to intensity of the braking manoeuvre. Upon the vehicle deceleration depends whether the rotating pedestrian will be on the bonnet, or in the case of braking of the vehicle—will fall before it.
- Roof vault—the situation in the first stage is similar to the somersault configuration, yet occurs at higher vehicle speeds or when the vehicle characterises a wedge (sports) design. The pedestrian is undercut by a vehicle, resulting in the body rotation. If the pedestrian is not in contact with the vehicle, the axis of rotation passes through the centre of mass of the pedestrian. In the next phase of accident pedestrian is shifted above the roof of the vehicle, and then falls behind the vehicle.
- Fender vault—the situation in which the pedestrian is struck by part of a corner of the car. The first contact points are the pedestrian's legs. Due to the proximity of the corner and bonnet edge, pedestrian falls over on the side of the vehicle.
- Dragging—the configuration of a collision in which a pedestrian, due to the primary impact, is dragged under the vehicle's chassis. Dragging a pedestrian under the vehicle can be characterised by accidents involving vehicles with a high bumper and high bonnet reference line. As a result of pulling the pedestrian's lower leg under the vehicle and its possible jamming, it becomes an instant centre of rotation of the pedestrian centre of mass.

It should be noted that the configuration depends primarily on the bumper and bonnet reference line relative to the pedestrian centre of mass. Thus, for a 5th-percentile woman the forward projection may occur during a collision with a standard compact vehicle. Conversely, the same scenario involving a 95th-percentile male pedestrian will likely result in wrap projection due to the higher pedestrian centre of mass. In view of the above, a collision with a small child and compact vehicle can be characterised by a similar configuration as the kinematic of a tall pedestrian (> 1.74 m) struck by a high bonnet vehicle such as SUV.

The configurations depicted in Fig. 4.2 are necessary to understand the causes of injuries that struck pedestrians. Nevertheless, the current type-approval tests (Nord-fjærn and Zavareh 2016) which use impactors do not represent a very important issue, upon pedestrian injuries, i.e. the complete kinematics of the pedestrian motion. It has been earlier noticed that the overall pedestrian kinematics response may vastly differ if the legform impactor hits a car with a high bumper (Kadali and Vedagiri 2016; Asaithambi et al. 2016).

Still in Fig. 4.2, the subsequent phases of the pedestrian forward projection are clearly visible. With the simultaneous presentation of the pedestrian and vehicle front-end, it can be easier to assess both the pedestrian kinematics and vehicle deformation.

The impact of a vehicle with a VRU has already been thoroughly studied and described in several publications, mainly through tests on human cadavers (Cesari et al. 1985; Kerrigan et al. 2012; Anderson et al. 2007) and increasingly popular testing on pedestrian dummies, carried out mainly in Japanese centres (Matsui et al. 2005; Yasuki and Yamamae 2010). The pedestrian and cyclist side impact test is the most commonly performed test since, according to Yang (2005) and Jarret and Saul (1998), it accounts for approximately 80% of VRU accidents, who are most often hit while crossing the road Jurecki and Stańczyk (2014).

Ravani et al. (1981), Kaeser and Devaud (1983), and later Ishikawa et al. (1994) and Mizuno and Kajzer (1999) addressed an issue known mainly from vehicle-to-vehicle collisions (O'Neill and Kyrychenko 2004), namely, that of the compatibility between vehicles and VRU. They stressed the influence of the geometry of mono-box vehicles on life-threatening injuries to the head, chest and abdomen. In the case of mono-box vehicles, injuries to these parts of the body are three times more frequent in comparison to compact vehicles with a clearly defined bonnet line. Figure 4.3 shows the head-to-bonnet impact carried out in Pam-Crash explicit code with Hybrid III modified-to-stand 50th percentile dummy impacted by a SUV front-end at 40 km/h. Unlike MADYMO pedestrian dummy—presented further—this developed dummy cannot be applied for lower extremities injury verification since none bone fracture joint switch or "add-erosion" card were implemented at this stage of research.

However, Fig. 4.3 presents the head impact situation, which is common in road accidents where VRU is involved. Head impacts are the most dangerous type of accidents and TBI is a major cause of death and disability worldwide, especially in children and young adults. Worldwide, an estimated 10 million people are affected annually by TBI (Gean and Fischbein 2010). Figure 4.4 illustrates the CT of a man in his fifties struck by a vehicle. It consists in an AIS5 level of injury, where skull

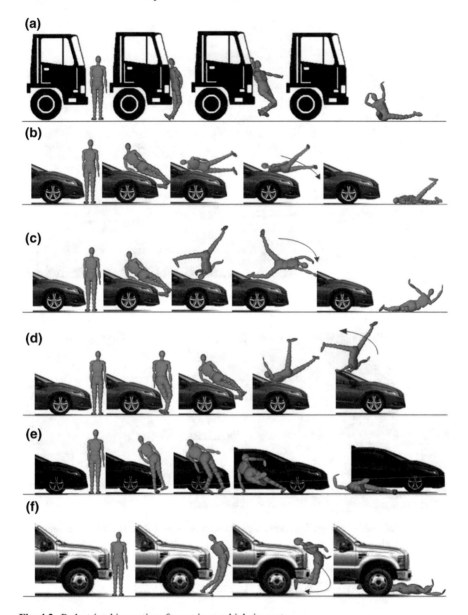

Fig. 4.2 Pedestrian kinematics after various vehicle impacts

bone fracture can be observed on the left side: parietal and temporal bone with the dislocation of fragments outside. Moreover, the skull base is fractured: temporal bone pyramid, left and sphenoid bone with visible blood in the sphenoidal.

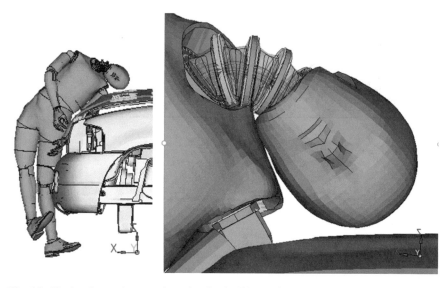

Fig. 4.3 Head-to-bonnet impact of a pedestrian in 100 ms after SUV-to-pedestrian accident at 40 km/h—numerical simulation with Hybrid III dummy (no lower extremities failure criteria)

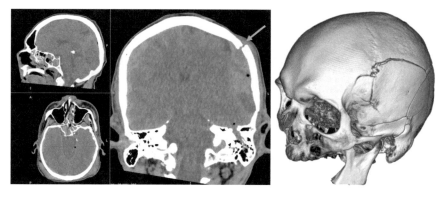

Fig. 4.4 CT of a male involved in a traffic accident with some visible skull fractures (courtesy of A. Kwiatkowski, MD)

4.3   Case Study—Pedestrian Accident Analysis

Computer simulations have been evolving concurrently with the rapid growth of advanced computers. Currently, their contribution to car design and safety devices process is vital. When the Finite Element Method—the already discussed technique used to determine the approximated solution for a partial differential equations on a defined domain—started to be used by appropriate software and powerful hardware, the complexities of modelling, including safety issues, could be addressed (Czmo-

$$[M]\{\ddot{r}\}_n + [C]\{\dot{r}\}_n + [K]\{r\}_n = \{F_{ext}\}_n$$

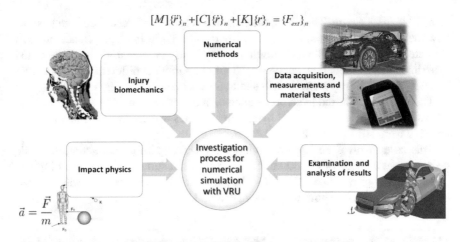

Fig. 4.5 Computer-aided forensic investigation model for vulnerable road user cases

chowski et al. 2014; Baranowski et al. 2014). Figure 4.5 depicts an authors' approach for forensic investigation where a vulnerable road user is involved.

The presented case is in fact a real-world accident, which has been chosen by the authors due to its importance in perspective of numerical analysis using both the finite element as well as multibody approaches. Lawsuits have been already investigated by many accident reconstructionists, experts and witnesses who were set up by various court instances. Nevertheless, the provided expertise is still contradictory as the case

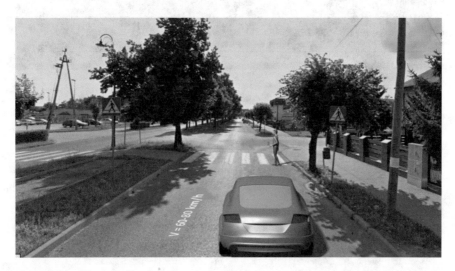

Fig. 4.6 The accident scene and a possible vehicle-pedestrian configuration—a visualisation in accordance with a witness testimony

is intricate in its nature. Therefore, the case was selected and described here to show how the numerical simulations can contribute not only in forensic science but also validate some hypothesis which would be very costly or even not ethic once tested experimentally. A numerical analysis can look at a variety of different factors in order to determine what may have contributed to the accident.

The accident occurred in an urban zone on a one-way road, with a speed limit of 50 km/h, where a male (1.75 m of height) in his fifties was crossing a road on a zebra crossing from left to right (Fig. 4.6).

This case involves an alleged Audi TT driver, supposedly impacting the male pedestrian at a speed of 60–80 km/h. The pedestrian suffered severe head injuries that eventually proved fatal (Fig. 4.7). The part of the accident scenario was reported by an eye-witness, to whom the court gave credit.

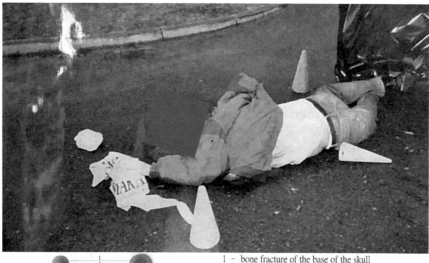

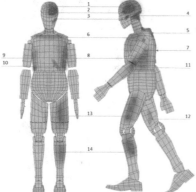

1 – bone fracture of the base of the skull
2 – brain injuries in the left lobe area
3 – fracture of the jaw bone on the left side
4 – rupture at the base of the skull
5 – injuries of the lower cervical and upper thoracic vertebrae
6 – broken clavicle
7 – rib fractures in the posterior plane, on the right side
8 – rib fractures in the lateral plane, on the left side
9 – rib fractures in the lateral plane, on the right side
10 – breaking of the rib arch
11 – injuries to the elbow
12 – wide hematoma distributed irregularly on the right thigh
13 – hip fracture on three levels
14 – fracture of tibia and fibula bone

Fig. 4.7 A victim of the accident—a man in his fifties at accident scene and the description of the injuries reported in post-mortem examination

However, the Audi TT driver claimed he did not strike the pedestrian. According to his testimony, the vehicle, which might have struck the man on pedestrian crossing was another car—Nissan Primera, which was driving on the left line, behind the Audi TT (Fig. 4.8).

Eventually, the Nissan Primera driver hit the tree just after the zebra crossing and the Audi TT driver drove away without stopping—reporting he did not realize that

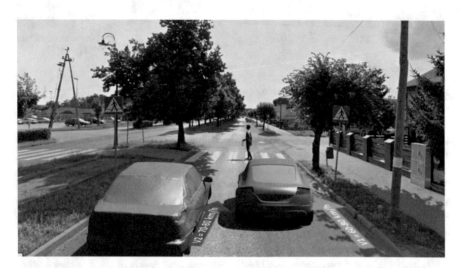

Fig. 4.8 A potential situation, where two vehicles were involved: Audi TT (right) and Nissan Primera (left)—a visualisation according to the Audi TT driver testimony

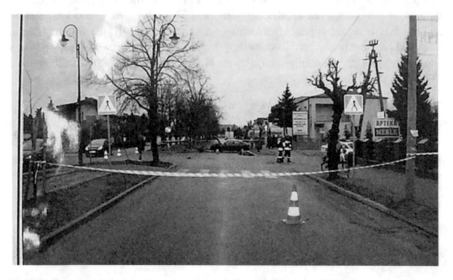

Fig. 4.9 An original photography presenting accident scene (Ptak et al. 2016)

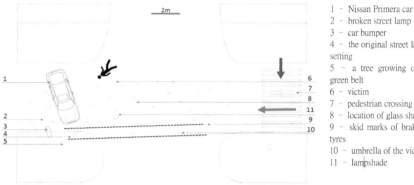

1 – Nissan Primera car
2 – broken street lamp
3 – car bumper
4 – the original street lamp setting
5 – a tree growing on a green belt
6 – victim
7 – pedestrian crossing
8 – location of glass shards
9 – skid marks of braking tyres
10 – umbrella of the victim
11 – lampshade

Fig. 4.10 Accident reconstruction drawing

any accident had happened. The accident scene is depicted in Fig. 4.9 and sketched in Fig. 4.10.

As the accident occurred in a small town, and there was presumably only one Audi TT car in the town, the witness indicated to the police officers the concrete suspected vehicle. The Audi TT was immediately found in the town by the police, confiscated and parked at the authorised parking lot as the proof of the case (Fig. 4.11). A young driver of Audi TT was eventually found guilty of causing the accident.

The presented hereinafter study is a numerical approach to evaluate a car-to-pedestrian accident from mechanical and biomechanical perspective. Another added-value of this work is to present the readers the level of plastic (permanent) deformation that may occur on the Audi TT 2007 numerical model, after impacting pedestrian dummy at the considered crash configurations. This may give a good estimation on how the car would appear after a collision. Correspondingly, the authors use the YEAHM previously depicted to show the possible head injuries of the pedestrian at a chosen possible impact configuration by the Nissan Primera. This approach required

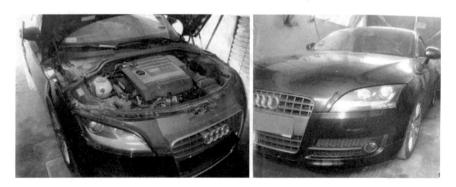

Fig. 4.11 The confiscated vehicle at the authorised parking lot right after the accident

some necessary steps including e.g. detailed vehicle measurements and constitutive modelling, to be presented hereafter.

4.3.1   Audi TT Vehicle Measurement

The CAD/CAE model of vehicles are rarely released, due to legal and know-how disclosure issues, by automotive companies or remodelled by some professional organisations such as National Crash Analysis Center of the George Washington University in the United States of America. Currently, there is no detailed FE model of Audi TT 2007. Thus, the authors needed to use reverse engineering method to create a 3D virtual model of an existing vehicle (Szelewski and Wieczorowski 2015). The physical object was measured using 3D scanning technologies.

The used laser scanner is 808 nm wavelength unit, which measures the distance using the interferometry technology. The head of scanner rotates in horizontal and vertical axis. The combination of two-axis rotation results in measurement of a spherical coordinate system. The interferometry is realized by Waveform Digitizing technology (WFD) where a processor calculates distances based on the time difference between reflected laser signal and referent signal. The precision of 3D point position is subjected to measurements distance as well as to the reflectivity of the scanned surface—precisely albedo or material reflectivity coefficient. A dedicated software such as Cyclon by Leica combines each of scanned cloud of point in spherical coordinate system to single common i.e. Cartesian coordinate system. The result of the measurement is a combined cloud of points from all scans, which is the basis for reproducing the geometry of the vehicle. The resulting point-to-point scanning tolerance was approximately 2 mm. Additionally, the scanner was able to make a set of spherical images in the visible light band which were further automatically mapped on the cloud of points. This feature enabled a photorealistic reproduction of a scanned object in three-dimensional space, which supports to interpret and work on the results in a CAD software.

The research included a total of four different vehicle scans and components to identify the geometry of the vehicle as complete as possible. The following objects were scanned:

1. The complete Audi TT vehicle with closed and open bonnet to reflect the outer geometry and the bonnet: Figs. 4.12 and 4.13:
2. The lifted Audi TT car with front bumper and head lights disassembled and open bonnet to 3D scan the vehicle front-end and normally hidden components (Figs. 4.14 and 4.15).
3. Detailed 3D scans of disassembled components such as a bonnet, bummer, headlights, which are especially important for proper vehicle-to-pedestrian numerical simulation (Fig. 4.16).

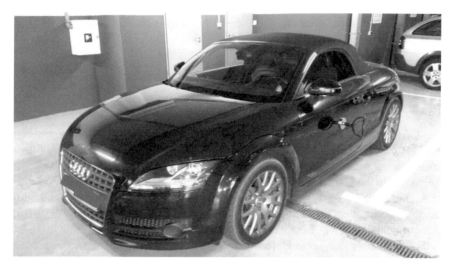

Fig. 4.12 3D scanning of the vehicle—first set up of a complete vehicle

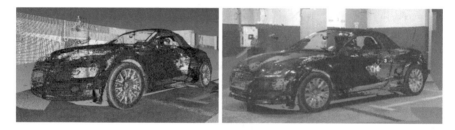

Fig. 4.13 The points of clouds of the vehicle—with the reflectivity colour spectrum (left) and spherical images mapped on the cloud of points (right)

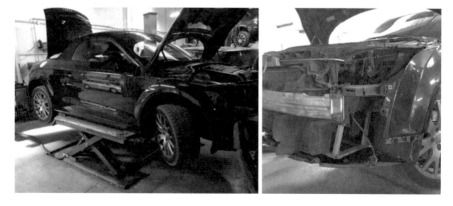

Fig. 4.14 3D scanning of the vehicle—second set up with disassembled components

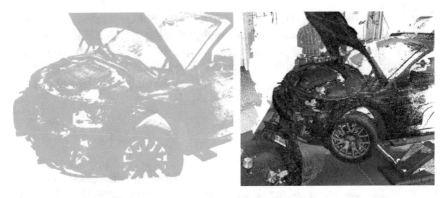

Fig. 4.15 The points of clouds from second set up—the exported cloud of points to a CAD software (left) and spherical images mapped on the cloud of points (right)

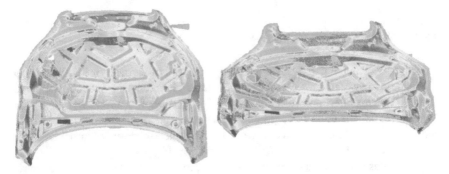

Fig. 4.16 The points of clouds from third set up—the scanned engine-side of the bonnet with the reflectivity colour spectrum

The result of the laser scan was an assembled point cloud including some detailed scanned components. In the next step, it was converted in CATIA V5 software. After filtering, the cloud of points was subjected to a triangulation process. Based on the triangle grid, NURBS (Non-Uniform Rational B-Spline) surfaces were generated. The result of geometry processing is a 3D solid-surface model.

4.3.2 Material Testing and Verification

From the perspective of pedestrian injuries and kinematics after a car impact, there are some crucial components, which material is required to be studied in detail. The authors disassembled and tested the bonnet, bonnet inner reinforcement, front bumper and other vehicle front-end components. The bonnet consists of two inter-connected parts—the outer metal sheet and the inner sheet, which is its reinforcing structure. Because of the pedestrian wrap-around distance (WAP), the bonnet and its reinforcement have a significant impact on pedestrian injuries during a crash (Ishikawa et al. 1993). In the first step in the study was the measurement of metal alloys by the use of an X-ray spectrometer.

4.3.2.1 X-Ray Spectrometer Tests

The measurements using the Bruker X-ray spectrometer are presented in Fig. 4.17. Basing on the measurements, the authors stated that the material used for the bonnet outer sheet is made of 6061 aluminium alloy and the AlMg2 aluminium alloy is used for the bonnet reinforcement.

4.3.2.2 Material Samples Testing

From the mechanical perspective, the most important properties for FE simulations are relations between true stress and true strain. Therefore, the second part of the research was to collect and verify mechanical properties of materials. For this task, a Zwick Roel 030 machine was used. From each tested element from the vehicle front-end, i.e. bonnet, bonnet reinforcement and front bumper (made of polypropylene with an admixture of elastomer) 4 samples were cut out (Fig. 4.18).

On the basis of static tensile test (Fig. 4.19), the engineering stress-strain curves are obtained. To get the true stress-strain values, the measured values should be

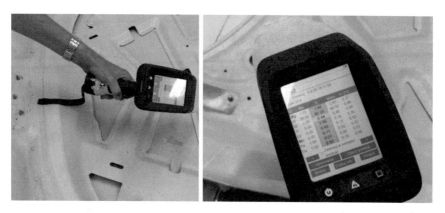

Fig. 4.17 The results of the bonnet measurements using X-ray spectrometer

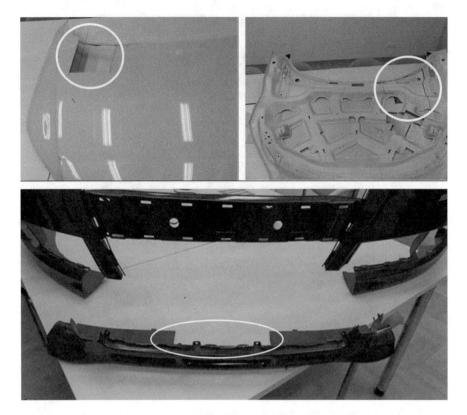

Fig. 4.18 Vehicle components—places are marked from which the samples were cut

converted according to mathematical formulas 4.1 and 4.2. In the area of small strain, engineering and true curves are covering each other. Divergences appear only with some greater strain.

$$\tilde{\sigma} = \sigma(1 + \varepsilon) \qquad (4.1)$$

$$\tilde{\varepsilon} = ln(1 + \varepsilon) \qquad (4.2)$$

where $\tilde{\sigma}$ is the true stress, σ is the engineering stress, ε is the engineering strain and $\tilde{\varepsilon}$ is the true strain.

The used FE software requires true stress-strain curves to be provided—the true stress-strain curves for the selected components are depicted in Fig. 4.20.

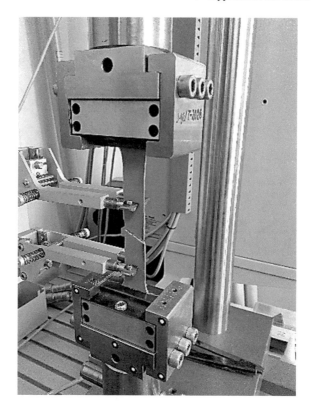

Fig. 4.19 Test of aluminium alloy specimen on the universal testing machine

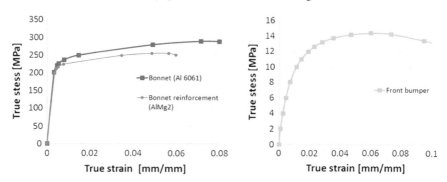

Fig. 4.20 True stress-strain curves for selected components

4.4 Finite Element Vehicle Model

Based on the obtained and processed 3D point cloud, the geometrical model of Audi TT was created in CATIA V5 and ICEM Surf software. The CAD model of the vehicle is depicted in Fig. 4.21.

Based on the developed geometric model of the Audi TT 2007 vehicle, a discrete model was created by applying the methodology, earlier validated for pedestrian accidents (Ptak et al. 2012; Kopczyński et al. 2011), namely:

- applying finite element mesh onto the vehicle CAD model: the average size of the shell type finite element stretched on the front of the vehicle was 10 mm.
- the application of a solid mesh to thick-wall elements (motor, battery, etc.) or these parts where a solid mesh is required, i.e. expanded polypropylene (EPP) energy-absorbing foam on the cross-beam at the front of the vehicle.
- applying 1D elements, i.e. a spring with appropriate stiffness to mimic the fastening of plastic clips and flexible joints; spotwelds where a glued connection (the bonnet with reinforcement) or a riveted one were required.
- modelling rigid connections (NASTRAN RBE2 element) between rigid components and the centre of mass of the vehicle—reflecting the centre of mass as a discrete element with a concentrated mass 1011 kg, with a total vehicle weight of 1405 kg.

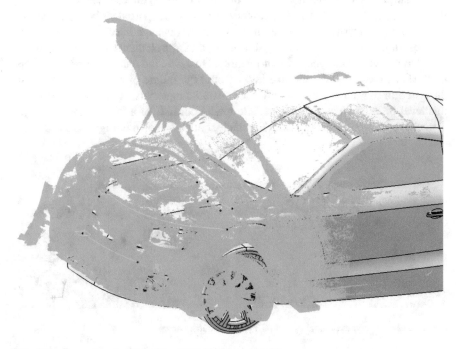

Fig. 4.21 Geometrical model of Audi TT 2007 based on 3D scan

The following material description models and contacts were used in LS-DYNA code (National Crash Analysis Center 2007; Ptak and Karliński 2012):

- *Piecewise linear plasticity*, elasto-plastic material with a stress-strain curve and strain rate dependency: bonnet, bonnet reinforcement, bumper, vehicle cover, rims, front lamps, other plastics;
- *Rigid*—ground;
- *Elastic*, an isotropic elastic material: tires;
- *Crushable foam*, material to model crushable foams with fully elastic unloading and elastic-perfectly-plastic tension at the tension cut-off threshold: energy-absorbing element behind the bumper (on the longitudinal beam) made of EPP 150 g/l;
- *Spring elastoplastic with damage*, the material which provides an elastoplastic translational spring with isotropic hardening with damage criterion: clips, plastic fasteners—stiffness k from 30 to 60 N/mm;
- The *automatic-general* contact algorithm was used with friction coefficient $\mu =$ 0.4–0.5 and *automatic surface-to-surface* with $\mu = 0.5$ at the bonnet contact and bonnet reinforcement.
- The *contact-coupling* to define the coupling surface for MADYMO to couple LS-DYNA—contact parameters set in MADYMO. This was required as the MADYMO pedestrian dummy model was used.

The automatic integration step, compatible (not larger) than MADYMO *coupling* was set. Due to the fact that during the pedestrian impact a partial yield of the material (material non-linearity) may occur and a significant change in configuration due to the large deflections (geometric non-linearity), all finite elements used are adapted to calculations with both types of non-linearity. However, the material models (except from 1D connections) do not take into account the failure of the material, because the criterion of failure, especially for non-metallic materials, is difficult to define at this level of detail. The discrete vehicle model consists of a total of 104255 finite elements and 106351 nodes. The FE vehicle model is shown in Figs. 4.22 and 4.23.

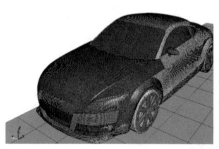 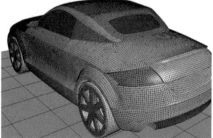

Fig. 4.22 Finite element model of Audi TT—axonometric views

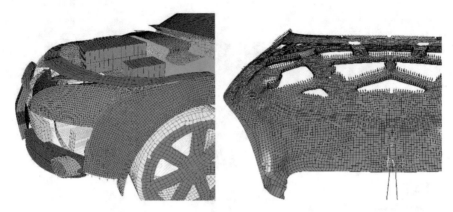

Fig. 4.23 Finite element model of Audi TT—a view without bumper and bonnet (left) and the bonnet reinforcement (right) with visible glue connections

4.5 MultiBody Dummy Model

The authors carried out multibody simulations using the MADYMO code. As the distinct from the FE, for the kinematic analysis evaluation there is no need to model detailed material characteristics. The geometry of the impacting body—i.e. the vehicle front-end—is the key factor for ensuring the pedestrian safety post-impact trajectory.

The use of the MADYMO dummy instead of the FE model enabled reducing the duration of the numerical calculations significantly. MADYMO contains advanced, well-developed and validated dummies; on the other hand, LS-DYNA provides accurate contact definitions and advanced materials models. An additional advantage of the process in the computational testing is time efficiency. Therefore, the use of the MADYMO Hybrid III 50th percentile pedestrian to simulate the kinematics of struck pedestrian and then reflect the boundary conditions on the FE advanced head model was considered a suitable solution.

It was decided to use an ellipsoidal pedestrian dummy from the MADYMO v7.5 library. This dummy is widely used in pedestrian safety tests and its biofidelity has been confirmed by numerous independent institutions (Anderson et al. 2007; Simms and Wood 2009; Lawrence et al. 2007; Stevenson 2006; Hoof et al. 2003). In addition, the FE dummy (e.g. the THUMS v4 model (Dyna More 2012)) introduces a number of parameters which are not essential for the correct representation of kinematics, and can introduce many complications into the calculations (Ishikawa et al. 1993; Pezowicz and Głowacki 2012). MADYMO dummies also do not require large computing power, which in view of the number of impact configurations was undoubtedly an advantage. The used dummy model in tests is the 50th-percentile male—depicted in its basic stance in Fig. 4.24.

Based on the results of tests (Stevenson 2006; Fricke 1990), the contact point between the dummy and the ground was defined as well as the appropriate coefficient

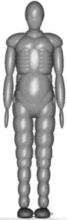

Height of standing dummy [m]	Shoulder width [m]	Knee height [m]	Dummy mass [kg]	The height of the centre of mass [m]
1.74	0.47	0.54	75.7	0.97

Fig. 4.24 Pedestrian dummy model used in the tests: MADYMO 50th-percentile male with its anthropometric data (Netherlands Organization for Applied Scientific Research 2011)

of friction between the soles of the dummy's shoes and the ground (asphalt concrete), equal to 0.55. The dummy was positioned in such a way that, at the point of contact with the vehicle model described below, the dummy's legs were loaded with the mass of the dummy, and its shoes were in contact with the ground. During the entire simulation, the dummy was in the field of acceleration $g = 9.81$ m/s^2.

4.6 Vehicle-to-Pedestrian Impact Configuration

During the course of a forensic investigation, it was concluded that the victim was standing on his left foot. This was evidenced by the left shoe's sole skid marks and grooves due to the sole-to-tarmac friction. Taking into consideration the pedestrian stances in which the reaction force acts only on the left foot (Simms and Wood 2009; Crocetta et al. 2015; Ramamurthy et al. 2011; Li et al. 2016) the authors defined the following accident configurations depicted in Fig. 4.25.

Further, some different pedestrian positions were established relative to the median longitudinal plane of the vehicle: Y = −0.2 m; −0.3 m; −0.62 m; −0.82 m; −0.88 m; −1.2 m in accordance with the coordinate system where point Y=0 lies on the median longitudinal plane of the vehicle (Fig. 4.26).

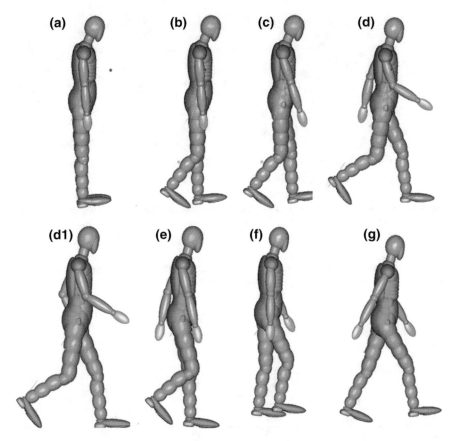

Fig. 4.25 The pedestrian stances (A-G) where the ground reaction force acts mainly on the left foot

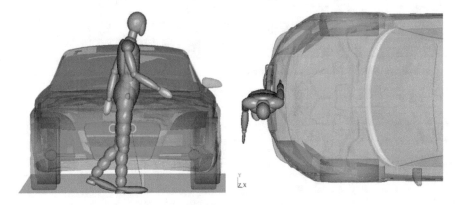

Fig. 4.26 An exemplary configuration Y = 0: front view (left), top view (right)

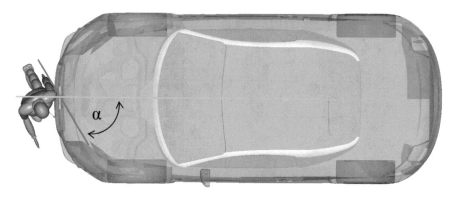

Fig. 4.27 The angle α [°] of the median plane of the dummy relative to the median longitudinal plane of the vehicle

Another variable was the angle α of the median plane (*planus medianum*) of the dummy relative to the median longitudinal plane of the vehicle, as illustrated in Fig. 4.27 .

In total, 19 crash configurations were analysed—parameters of which are presented in Table 4.1.

Table 4.1 Impact configuration matrix

Configuration no.	Dummy Y position [m]	Angle α [°]	Dummy stance	Vehicle velocity at impact (V_0) [km/h]
1	−0.62	90	A	80
2	−0.82	90	B	80
3	−0.82	90	C	50
4	−0.82	90	C	70
5	−0.82	90	C	60
6	−0.82	90	C	80
7	−0.82	90	D	80
8	−0.82	90	D	75
9	−0.82	90	D	70
10	−1.2	90	D	75
11	−1.2	90	D	65
12	−0.2	90	D	75
13	−0.82	90	D1	75
14	−0.3	90	D1	75
15	−0.82	90	E	75
16	−0.62	90	E	75
17	−0.82	90	F	75
18	−0.88	90	G	60
19	−0.62	80	D1	60

4.7 Analysis of the Results

Due to the complexity of numerical simulations and crash configurations, the authors presented only the most important time-windows of the three most representative analysis, more specifically the configurations 3rd (Figs. 4.28 and 4.29), 14th (Figs. 4.30 and 4.31) and 19th (Figs. 4.32 and 4.33). The attention was focused on structural elements that are permanently (plastically—e.g.: bonnet dent) deformed after impact with a pedestrian. Thus, these damaged outer vehicle components would be easily noticeable for the police officers and an expert witness during the vehicle inspection after the car was officially confiscated. Further, some of the damage components would be noticeable on the official pictures taken after the accident. The results of individual crash configurations are presented in Figs. 4.28, 4.29, 4.30, 4.31, 4.32 and 4.33.

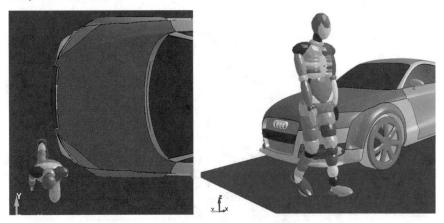

Fig. 4.28 Impact configuration no. 3—top view (left) and axonometric view (right)

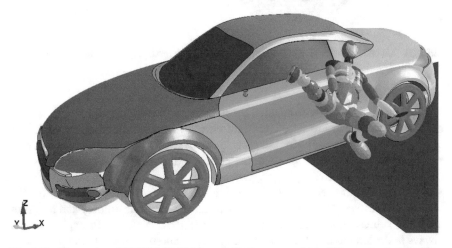

Fig. 4.29 Kinematics of MADYMO 50th percentile dummy model in 200 ms after impact (configuration no. 3)

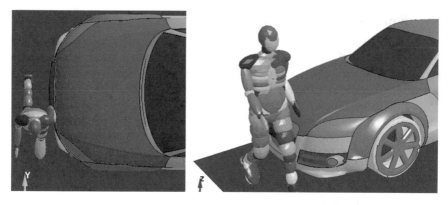

Fig. 4.30 Impact configuration no. 14—top view (left) and axonometric view (right)

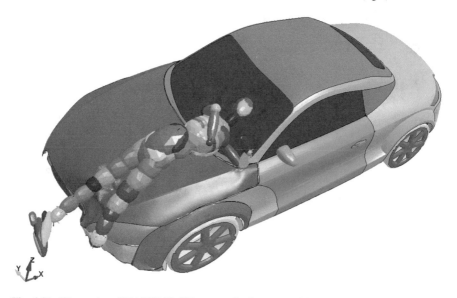

Fig. 4.31 Kinematics of MADYMO 50th percentile dummy model in 86 ms after impact (configuration no. 14)

The commenced analysis enabled the authors to have an insight into the vehicle deformation after the impact. Figure 4.34 clearly illustrates the level of permanent deformation (plastic strain) for the representative configurations. In order to better visualise the front-end deformation, the plastic strain level was set in the range of 0.001/0.1 (i.e.: 0.1%/10%).

As a result of the performed numerical tests, the authors concluded that for the considered crash configurations, using a numerical pedestrian dummy and the Audi TT 2007 vehicle model, significant (more than 10%) plastic deformation occurs always in the structure of the front bumper, fender and/or bonnet. These permanent deformations shall be clearly visible on the vehicle.

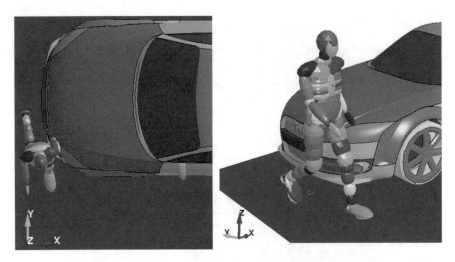

Fig. 4.32 Impact configuration no. 19—top view (left) and axonometric view (right)

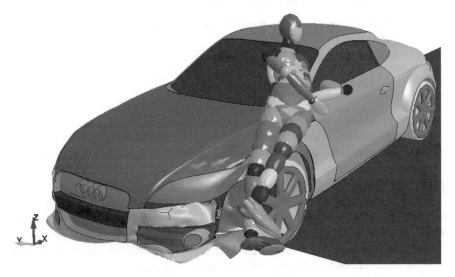

Fig. 4.33 Kinematics of MADYMO 50th percentile dummy model in 83 ms after impact (configuration no. 19)

It is noted that this report is not to be regarded as an official reconstruction of a road accident—as this have been done already by five independent experts in collision and trajectory simulation software such as PC-Crash and V-SIM. However, these reports are contradictory. Thus, this work is an approach to present the level of plastic deformation (permanent) that occurs on an Audi TT 2007 vehicle, after striking a pedestrian dummy in regard to a particular, considered collision configuration.

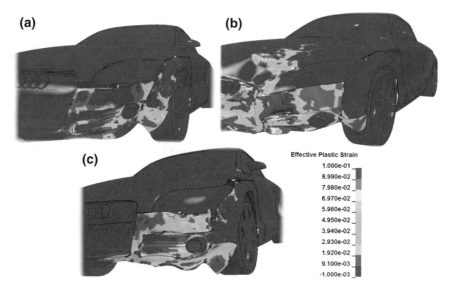

Fig. 4.34 Effective plastic strain map [mm/mm] on the vehicle in 83 ms after the impact for configuration no. 3 (**a**); 14 (**b**); 19 (**c**)

4.8   Head to Windshield Impact

This section depicts an approach to simulate the hypothetical case where the Nissan Primera was involved in the pedestrian accident. This possibility was finally rejected by the court, mainly because it was in contrast with the eyewitness testimony. The eyewitness indicated the Audi TT vehicle as the one, which impacted the pedestrian on the zebra crossing. Incidentally, the psychologist Schacter (1999) summarised the common flaws of human memory and noted in his publication "The seven sins of memory" the tendency to form false memories. Human memories, unlike computer algorithm, tend to operate through association and activity of memory networks. Although this system of memorising is very quick, it is subjected to many myriad vulnerabilities. Therefore, psychologist advocate treat eye-witness testimony with more suspicion than is the case in most courts in the world (Jarrett 2015).

Thus, the possibility of Nissan Primera-to-pedestrian impact was auxiliary investigated by the authors and the research is presented hereinafter. The photographic documentation of Nissan Primera after the accident is still accessible (Ptak et al. 2016) and part of the documentation is illustrated in Fig. 4.35.

The damages on Nissan Primera front-end are similar to these reported in the literature for a pedestrian warp projection, a car accident involving pedestrians and compact cars, head injuries occur very frequently as the head of the pedestrian hits the windshield. This is caused because of the geometrical proportion of a pedestrian and vehicle's front end i.e. WAD. For instance, the damages on Nissan Primera front-end are similar to these reported in the literature for a pedestrian warp projection

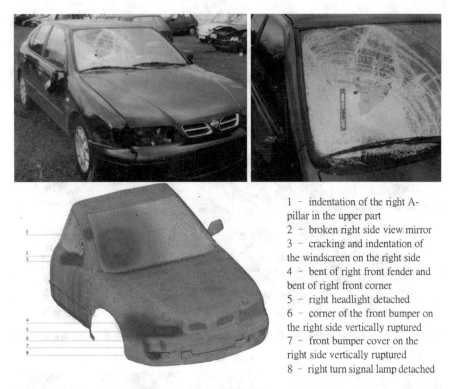

1 – indentation of the right A-pillar in the upper part
2 – broken right side view mirror
3 – cracking and indentation of the windscreen on the right side
4 – bent of right front fender and bent of right front corner
5 – right headlight detached
6 – corner of the front bumper on the right side vertically ruptured
7 – front bumper cover on the right side vertically ruptured
8 – right turn signal lamp detached

Fig. 4.35 The damages of Nissan Primera front-end (Ptak et al. 2016)

(Ptak et al. 2012; Simms and Wood 2009). Comparable vehicle damages, as for Nissan Primera, were observed in an unmarked police car (Dodge Charger shown in Fig. 4.36), which fatally struck a pedestrian at about 65 km/h (Toohey 2003).

4.8.1 Geometry Acquisition

Unlike for the Audi TT model, where a 3D scanner was used, the outer geometry of the Nissan Primera was obtained by photogrammetric analysis. Comparing to 3D scanning, this is a low-cost and more accessible method. On the other hand, 3D reconstruction of geometry using pictures is considered as less accurate than obtained by high quality 3D scanners. Photogrammetry consists of compiling a set of 2D photographs of the object taken from different locations to generate 3D geometrical data. The vehicle model was generated in Autodesk ReCAP basing on 230 photographs taken in three perspectives, with approximately 10° of offset angle. The photographs were adjusted with manual white balance. The ReCAP software considered the camera positioning relative to the location of matched key features, used

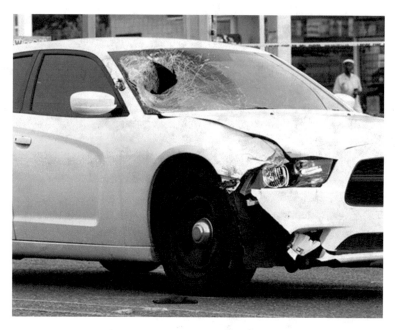

Fig. 4.36 The example of damages on Dodge Charger vehicle due to pedestrian strike at 65 km/h (Toohey 2003)

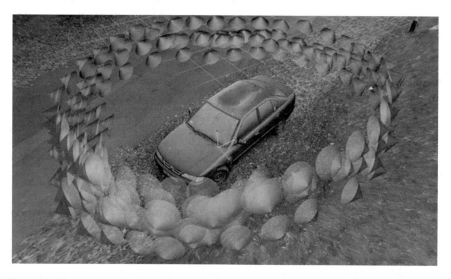

Fig. 4.37 Photorealistic model of Nissan Primera with marked places of taken photographs

as markers, on the object in different photographs (James et al. 2017). The obtained photorealistic model of the vehicle contained 4.5 million of triangles (Fig. 4.37).

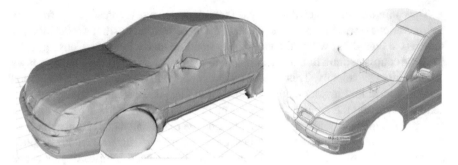

Fig. 4.38 Geometrical models of Nissan Primera front-end: stereolithographic (left) and surface model (right)

The STL model was further converted into geometrical model using NURBS mathematical model to represent the curves and surfaces (Fig. 4.38). The generated CAD model was further utilised in FEA simulations. Hereby, the authors also proved that the photogrammetry is a robust method to obtain vehicle outer geometry—especially in situations where the use of 3D scanner is limited.

4.8.2 Boundary Conditions

The simulation of a vehicle collision with a pedestrian dummy model was carried out based on two numerical codes (LS-DYNA and MADYMO) coupled with each other. The coupling of both programs made it possible to carry out a full analysis of the collision of a vehicle with the pedestrian. The MADYMO pedestrian model was the same, 50th percentile male, as in the Audi TT case.

The aim of the carried out simulations was to investigate the kinematics of struck pedestrian to mimic the windshield damages presented in Fig. 4.35. The front-end model of the Nissan Primera was not tested thoroughly comparing to the described Audi TT due to lack of physical components. Therefore, the generic stiffness, basing on similar age vehicle—i.e. Dodge Neon (National Crash Analysis Center 1996)—was established in the numerical model. However, the state-of-the-art is that to reflect the overall pedestrian kinematics of a struck pedestrian where the geometry plays a crucial role, not the front-end stiffness which is an order of magnitude higher than human's body stiffness (Simms et al. 2015; Simms and Wood 2009). However, to reflect biomechanics of the head, which apparently impacted the vehicle's windshield, the authors needed its accurate model. Thus, particular attention was drown to model the Nissan Primera windshield precisely, by a method which will be introduced in next pages of this book.

   The configuration depicted in Fig. 4.39 was chosen as most representative from the configurations tested (Wrzeszcz et al. 2017). The pedestrian positions reflect the D1 stance (see Figs. 4.25) where the victim was standing on his left foot. Consequently, from the coupled simulation it was possible to obtain the orientation of the dummy's head and its CG velocity. This data became the boundary condition for the detailed head-to-windshield impact using the YEAHM. This assessment of the severity of head injury using the advanced FE head model was performed in Abaqus explicit code as both the head and the windshield model were validated under this numerical code. The following paragraph describes the necessary steps undertaken to complete the final head-to-windshield simulation and verify the head injuries of the struck pedestrian.

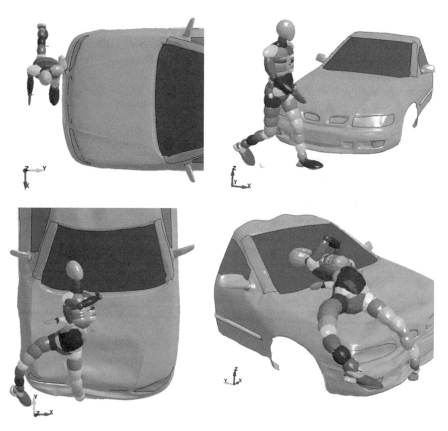

Fig. 4.39 Impact configuration with Nissan Primera (top row) and kinematics of MADYMO 50th percentile dummy model in 94 ms after the impact—the moment when the head touches the windshield (lower row)

4.8.3 Windshield Modeling

In particular, the type of windshield used in this study is a polyvinyl butyral (PVB) laminated windshield. PVB keeps the glass layers bonded even after glass failure, preventing it from breaking into large sharp pieces. Therefore, the glass determines the behaviour of the windshield for small deformations, while for large deformations the PVB layer plays a dominant role.

The FE windshield model was modelled in Abaqus 6.12-3 explicit code. All the three windshield layers were modelled with shell elements, projecting the geometry of a real windshield from a production car. The four-node and three-node shell elements available in Abaqus were used (Abaqus' S4 and S3 elements, respectively). An illustration of this three layered structure is shown in Fig. 4.40. The glass shell layers are tied to the PVB shell layer, assuming the full bonding between the glass and the PVB interlayer.

PVB was modelled as a hyperelastic material with Ogden's potential. This model was used to describe the nonlinear stress-strain behaviour of PVB. The Ogden strain energy function is defined by:

$$\tilde{U} = \sum_{i=1}^{N} \frac{2\mu_i}{\alpha_i^2} (\bar{\lambda}_1^{\alpha_i} + \bar{\lambda}_2^{\alpha_i} + \bar{\lambda}_3^{\alpha_i} - 3) + \sum_{i=1}^{N} \frac{1}{D_i} (J^{el} - 1)^{2i} \tag{4.3}$$

where the deviatoric principal stretches are computed by $\bar{\lambda}_i = J^{-\frac{1}{3}}\lambda_i$, λ_i are the principal stretches, N, μ_i, α_i and D_i are material parameters. The initial shear modulus and bulk modulus are given by:

$$\mu_0 = \sum_{i=1}^{N} \mu_i \tag{4.4}$$

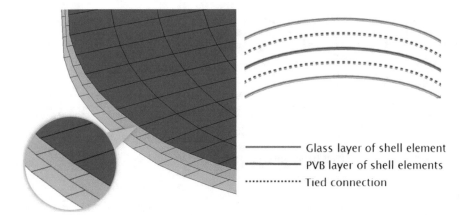

Glass layer of shell element
PVB layer of shell elements
Tied connection

Fig. 4.40 Windshield mesh (left) and its 3-tied structure (right)

Table 4.2 Post failure stress-strain relation values

Direct stress after cracking [MPa]	Direct cracking strain
120	0
0	1E-5

$$K_0 = \frac{2}{D_1} \tag{4.5}$$

More details about the rubber-like behaviour that describes this material law, based on stretches, can be found in Ogden (1972). The experimental data from the uniaxial tensile tests performed by Bennison et al. (2005) were used to fit the Ogden strain energy function of order 3. Figure 4.41 shows the stress-strain curve used in this work to characterise the material behaviour. In addition, the material was considered isotropic with a density of 1.1×10^3 kg/m^3 and Poisson's ratio (v) of 0.45.

In order to model the glass, the brittle cracking material model was used. It allows the removal of elements based on a brittle failure criterion. In order to define when the material cracks and the behaviour after crack initiation, three stages must be defined: a post failure stress-strain relation, a shear retention model and a brittle failure criterion. Table 4.2 shows the values used to define the post failure relation.

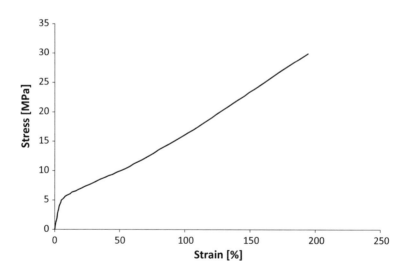

Fig. 4.41 Behaviour of PVB (Bennison et al. 2005)

Table 4.3 Shear retention model values

ρ	e_{nn}^{ck}
1	0
0.5	1E-6

Regarding the shear retention model, Abaqus requires the definition of the post cracked shear stiffness as a function of the opening strain across the crack. This relation is defined by:

$$G_c = \rho(e_{nn}^{ck})G \tag{4.6}$$

where e_{nn}^{ck} is the strain after cracking, ρ is the shear retention factor and G_c is the cracked shear modulus. Table 4.3 shows the values used in this study for glass.

The material cracking is defined by a Rankine criterion based on the maximum stress to crack. One material point was set as requirement for element failure with a direct cracking failure strain of 0.002. Regarding glass linear elastic properties: Young's modulus of 74 GPa and Poisson's ratio of 0.227.

This windshield model is validated. Figure 4.42 shows the comparison between the windshield FE model crack pattern and the experimental crack pattern from van Rooij et al. (2003) experiments. There is a good agreement between simulations and experiments.

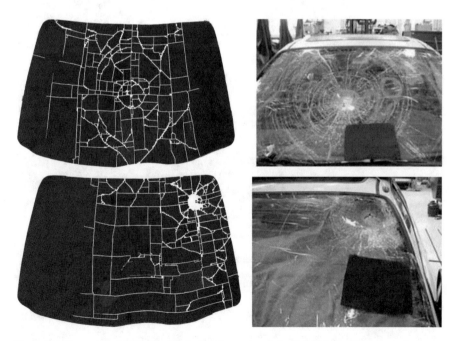

Fig. 4.42 Comparison between numerical and experimental windshield crack patterns for centre and corner impact positions: centre (top) and corner (bottom)

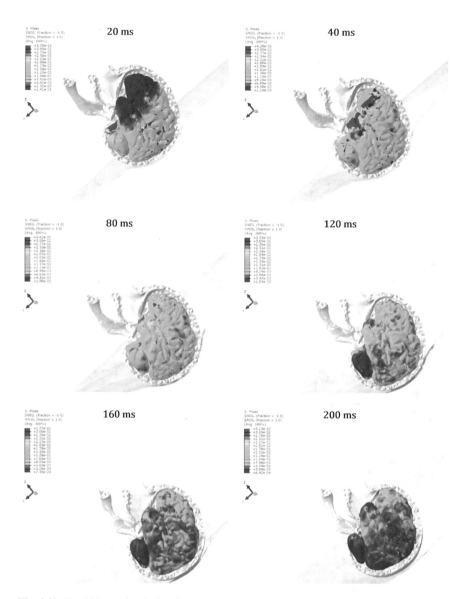

Fig. 4.43 Head kinematics during the windshield impact at 72 km/h—H-M-H stress map [MPa]

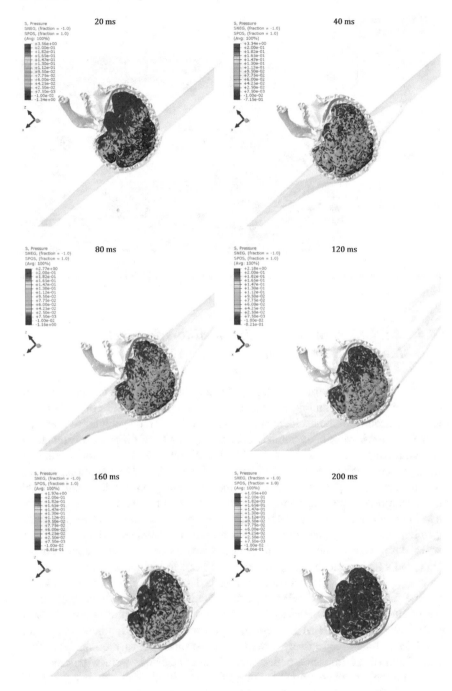

Fig. 4.44 Head kinematics during the windshield impact at 72 km/h—hydrostatic pressure [MPa]

S, Max. Principal
SPOS, (fraction = 1.0)
(Avg: 100%)

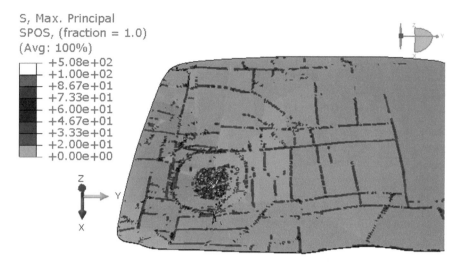

Fig. 4.45 Windshield at 200ms after impact—the crack pattern of PVB laminated glass, principal stress map [MPa]

4.8.4   Analysis of the Results for Head-to-Windshield Impact—Biomechanical Perspective

Reconstruction of pedestrian accidents using FE dummy models can be very time-consuming in terms of finding a correlation between the kinematics of the body and the information from the accident such as impact location on vehicle front-end and victim's injuries. Multibody models and FE models have different advantages in accident reconstructions, which were already mentioned in the previous paragraph. The approach of the authors was to carry out many multibody simulations to determine the setup and then apply the final match—basing on accident photographic documentation and post mortem examination—to the FE head model. Thus, basing on MADYMO dummy's head velocity run the authors read maximum vertical velocity to implement the boundary conditions for the simulations in Abaqus FEA. The vertical component of the head initial velocity was 72 km/h. The horizontal component (head's tangential velocity) was neglected due to kinematics of the pedestrian and the specific impact mechanism. The results depicted in Figs. 4.43 and 4.44 show the time frames of the YEAHM impacting the Nissan Primera windshield in the form of Huber-von Mises-Hencky (H-M-H) stress and hydrostatic pressure in brain, respectively. The brain H-M-H stress and hydrostatic pressure gradients depicted in Figs. 4.43 and 4.44 respectively, reveal the worst outcome: severe injuries that led to the death of the impacted pedestrian. These conclusions were withdrawn after comparing the results computed for these two variables with the injury thresholds presented in Tables 1.3 and 1.4 previously introduced (Chap. 1). Almost all the thresholds in these tables were exceeded. In addition, the numerical simulations allowed the authors to investigate the effect of the glass failure stress on the windshield model's behaviour (Fig. 4.45). Although the in-depth research is needed to model an actual windshield of a vehicle, this approach is fruitful for accident reconstructions.

4.9 Conclusions

Numerical models based on advanced, validated dummy models are now, along with tests on human cadavers and specialized physical pedestrian dummies, one of the most accurate ways to simulate vehicle-pedestrian collisions. In vehicle-to-pedestrian accidents, head injuries are one of the most common injury types and can lead to lifelong disability or death. A number of publications noted that brain deformation or strain is a principal mechanism of injury. However, measuring strain, especially in vivo, during an impact is a big challenge which also implies ethical issues. Thus, numerical simulations allow the authors to verify, among the others, vehicle deformation, pedestrian kinematics and head injury lever after a collision. The most robust methods are the finite element and multibody methods.

Nowadays, the aim of the study was to analyse the kinematic and injures of impacted pedestrian in various, potential impact configurations. The set of simulations were carried out to represent probable cases of a real-world accident. The level of details needed to simulate the vehicle-to-pedestrian impact requires to take a number of actions—e.g. the measurements of vehicle's geometric were taken by 3D laser scanner and photogrammetry method. The material data was derived from physical objects which allowed the numerical code to simulate the actual behaviour of the components of the vehicle and apply YEAHM for head injuries verification.

A new FEHM was here developed and validated against impacts performed on cadavers. YEAHM has a geometric accurate brain model with sulci and gyri structures, which can relative move to the skull. This work also shows the importance of a careful choice of finite element formulations to model body parts, especially the ones constituted by incompressible materials.

A good understanding of the injury mechanism is of uttermost importance when studying injury prevention. Without knowing the proper injury mechanism, the associated injury criteria and thresholds, it is not possible to use a FEHM to predict the type, location, and severity of a TBI. Validated, accurate and advanced FEHMs can be used in accident reconstructions, design of protective head gear and injury evaluation. Nevertheless, further validation against other experiments available in the literature is also a future objective.

It is emphasised that the results of the presented research are not an attempt to artistic presentation of the accident (visualisation, animation, image rendering), yet the physical representation of dynamic phenomena. The authors presented the excessive potential of computer-aided engineering and described the various numerical approaches for kinematics and head injury verification from biomechanical perspective. Furthermore, the presented methodology may be very useful to analyse other types of traumatic events occurring in contact sports or work accidents.

References

R.W.G. Anderson, L.D. Streeter, G. Ponte, J. McLean, Mc: pedestrian reconstruction using multi-body madymo simulation and the polar-li dummy: a comparison of head kinematics. ESV-Paper no. 07–0273, 1–15 (2007)

G. Asaithambi, M.O. Kuttan, S. Chandra, Pedestrian road crossing behavior under mixed traffic conditions: a comparative study of an intersection before and after implementing control measures. Transp. Dev. Econ. **2**, 14 (2016)

P. Baranowski, K. Damaziak, J. Malachowski, L. Mazurkiewicz, A. Muszyński, *A child seat numerical model validation in the static and dynamic work conditions* (Arch. Civ. Mech, Eng, 2014)

S. Bennison, J. Sloan, D. Kistunas, P. Buehler, T. Amos, C. Smith, *Laminated glass for blast mitigation: role of interlayer properties*. In: Glass processing days (2005)

D. Cesari, C. Cavallero, J. Farisse, J. Bonnoit, Effects of crash conditions on pedestrian leg kinematics and injuries based on cadaver and dummy tests, in *29th Annual Conference of The American Association For Automotive Medicine*, Washington D.C. (1985), pp. 275–285

G. Crocetta, S. Piantini, M. Pierini, C. Simms, The influence of vehicle front-end design on pedestrian ground impact. Accid. Anal. Prev. **79**, 56–69 (2015)

J. Czmochowski, P. Moczko, P. Odyjas, D. Pietrusiak, Tests of rotary machines vibrations in steady and unsteady states on the basis of large diameter centrifugal fans. Eksploat. i Niezawodn. **16**, 211–216 (2014)

Dyna More, Human Model—Total HUman Model for Safety THUMS v 4.0, (2012), http://www.dynamore.de/en/products/models/human-11/05/12

European Commission, Road safety in the European Union—Trends, statistics and main challenges (2015)

L.B. Fricke, Traffic Accident Reconstruction. Traffic Accid. Investig. **2**, (1990)

A.D. Gean, N.J. Fischbein, Head trauma. Neuroimaging Clin. N. Am. **20**, 527–56 (2010)

J. Hoof, R. de Lange, J.S.H.M. Wismans, Improving pedestrian safety using numerical human models. Stapp Car Crash J. **47**, 401–436 (2003)

H. Ishikawa, J. Kajzer, K. Ono, M. Sakurai, Simulation of car impact to pedestrian lower extremity: influence of different car-front shapes and dummy parameters on test results. Accid. Anal. Prev. **26**, 231–242 (1994)

H. Ishikawa, J. Kajzer, G. Schroeder, Computer simulation of impact response of the human body in car-pedestrian accidents. SAE Tech. Pap. 933129 (1993)

D.W. James, F. Belblidia, J.E. Eckermann, J. Sienz, An innovative photogrammetry color segmentation based technique as an alternative approach to 3D scanning for reverse engineering design. Comput. Aided. Des. Appl. **14**, 1–16 (2017)

C. Jarrett, *Great myths of the brain* (Wiley, New York, 2015)

K. Jarret, R. Saul, Pedestrian injury-analysis of the PCDS field collision data, in *Proceedings of the 16th International Enhanced Safety Vehicle Conference* (1998), pp. 1204–1211

R.S. Jurecki, T.L. Stańczyk, Driver reaction time to lateral entering pedestrian in a simulated crash traffic situation. Transp. Res. Part F Traffic Psychol. Behav. **27**, 22–36 (2014)

B.R. Kadali, P. Vedagiri, Proactive pedestrian safety evaluation at unprotected mid-block crosswalk locations under mixed traffic conditions. Saf. Sci. **89**, 94–105 (2016)

R. Kaeser, J. Devaud, Design aspects of energy absorption in car pedestrian impacts. SAE Tech. Pap. **830625**, 239–253 (1983)

J.R. Kerrigan, A.-D. Carlos, J. Foster, J.R. Crandall, A. Rizzo, Pedestrian injury analysis: field data versus laboratory experiments, in *IRCOBI Conference* **2012**, 672–689 (2012)

A. Kopczyński, M. Ptak, P. Harnatkiewicz, The influence of frontal protection system design on pedestrian passive safety. Arch. Civ. Mech. Eng. **11**, 345–364 (2011)

K. Fabian, A European Roadmap for cycling—ECF proposal. Eur. Cyclists' Fed. (2015)

G.J.L. Lawrence, I.M. Knight, I.C.P. Simmons, J.A. Carroll, G. Coley, R.S. Bartlett, A study of possible future developments of methods to protect pedestrians and other vulnerable road users. Project Report, UPR/VE/05/17.01 (2007)

G. Li, D. Otte, J. Yang, C. Simms, Can a small number of pedestrian impact scenarios represent the range of real-world pedestrian injuries, in *IRCOBI Conf. 2016* IRC-16-12 (2016)

Y. Matsui, A. Wittek, M. Tanahashi, Pedestrian kinematics due to impacts by various passenger cars using full-scale dummy. Int. J. Veh. Saf. **1**, 64 (2005)

K. Mizuno, J. Kajzer, Compatibility problems in frontal, side, single car collisions and car-to-pedestrian accidents in Japan. Accid. Anal. Prev. **31**, 381–391 (1999)

National Crash Analysis Center, *Finite Element Model of Dodge Neon FE Model of Dodge Neon* (The George Washington University, Washington D.C, 1996)

National Crash Analysis Center, *Finite Element Model of Ford F250* (The George Washingtion University, Washington D.C, 2007)

Netherlands Organization for Applied Scientific Research TNO: Human Models Manual. Madymo Release 7.4. TNO (2011)

T. Nordfjærn, M.F. Zavareh, Individualism, collectivism and pedestrian safety: a comparative study of young adults from Iran and Pakistan. Saf. Sci. **87**, 8–17 (2016)

B. O'Neill, S. Kyrychenko, Crash incompatibilities between cars and light trucks: issues and potential countermeasures. Veh. Aggress. Compat. Automot. Crashes, SAE SP-1878. **1**, 1829–1841 (2004)

R.W. Ogden, Large deformation isotropic elasticity: on the correlation of theory and experiment for incompressible rubberlike solids. Proc. R. Soc. Lond. A **326**, 565–584 (1972)

C. Pezowicz, M. Głowacki, The mechanical properties of human ribs in young adult. Acta Bioeng. Biomech. **12**, 53–60 (2012)

V. Podvezko, H. Sivilevičius, The use of AHP and rank correlation methods for determining the significance of the interaction between the elements of a transport system having a strong influence on traffic safety. Transport. **28**, 389–403 (2013)

M. Ptak, J. Karliński, Pedestrian passive safety during the SUV impact: regulations vs. reality, in *2012 IRCOBI Conf. Dublin, Irel* (2012), pp. 103–113

M. Ptak, E. Rusiński, J. Karliński, S. Dragan, E. Rusinski, J. Karlinski, S. Dragan, Evaluation of kinematics of SUV to pedestrian impact–Lower leg impactor and dummy approach. Arch. Civ. Mech. Eng. **12**, 68–73 (2012)

M. Ptak, E. Rusiński, M. Wnuk, J. Wilhelm, J. Wickowski, Numerical simulation using finite element method and mulitbody pedestrian dummy. Report no. 142/2016, Wroclaw (2016)

P. Ramamurthy, M.V. Blundell, C. Bastien, Y. Zhang, Computer simulation of real-world vehicle-pedestrian impacts. Int. J. Crashworthiness **16**, 351–363 (2011)

B. Ravani, D. Brougham, R.T. Mason, Pedestrian post-impact kinematics and injury patterns. Traffic Saf. P-97, 791–824 (1981)

D.L. Schacter, The seven sins of memory: Insights from psychology and cognitive neuroscience. Am. Psychol. **54**, 182–203 (1999)

C. Simms, D. Wood, *Pedestrian and Cyclist Impact* (Springer, Netherlands, Dordrecht, 2009)

C.K. Simms, D. Wood, R. Fredriksson, Pedestrian injury biomechanics and protection, in *Accidental Injury* (Springer, New York, 2015), pp. 721–753

T. Stevenson, Simulation of vehicle-pedestrian interaction, Dr. thesis (2006)

Supreame Audit Office in Poland, Cyclist and pedestrian safety. KIN.410.008.00.2015 (2016)

M. Szelewski, M. Wieczorowski, Reverse engineering and discretization methods of physical objects. Mechanik 976/183-976/188 (2015)

G. Toohey, Unmarked Baton Rouge police car strikes, kills pedestrian on florida street tuesday, http://www.theadvocate.com/baton_rouge/news/crime_police/. Accessed 01 Mar 2018

World Health Organization, Global status report on road safety. Inj. Prev. 318 (2015)

L. van Rooij, K. Bhalla, M. Meissner, J. Ivarsson, J. Crandall, D. Longhitano, Y. Takahashi, Y. Dokko, Y. Kikuchi, Pedestrian crash reconstruction using multi-body modeling with geometrically detailed, validated vehicle models and advanced pedestrian injury criteria, in *Proceedings of the 18th ESV Conference 468*, (Nagoya, 2003)

M. Wrzeszcz, M. Małolepszy, M. Ptak, *The approach to pedestrian impact analysis and accident reconstruction—thesis supervised by M* (Ptak. Wrocław Univeristy Sci, Technlogy, 2017)

J. Yang, Review of injury biomechanics in car-pedestrian collisions. Int. J. Veh. Saf. **1**, 100 (2005)

T. Yasuki, Y. Yamamae, Validation of kinematics and lower extremity injuries estimated by total human model for safety in suv to pedestrian impact test. J. Biomech. Sci. Eng. **5**, 340–356 (2010)